Recent Advances in Asthma Research and Treatments

Edited by Svetlana P. Chapoval

Published in London, United Kingdom

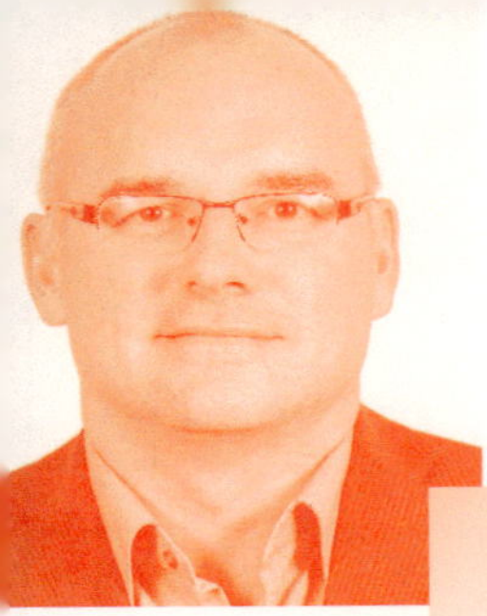
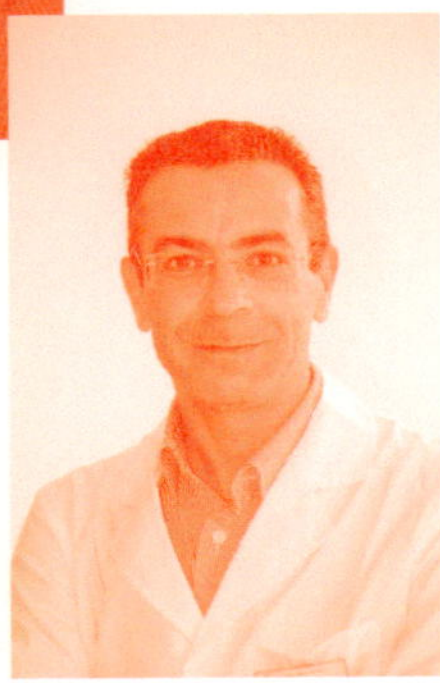
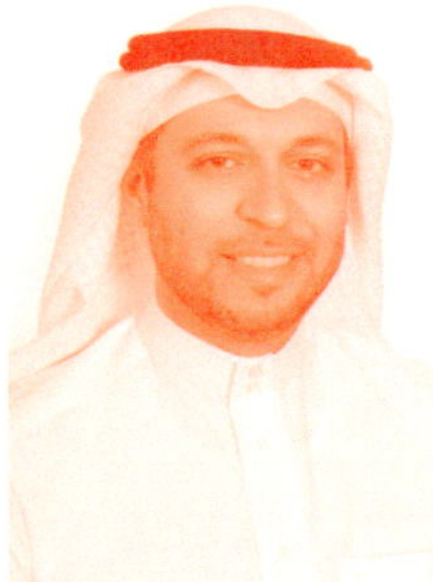
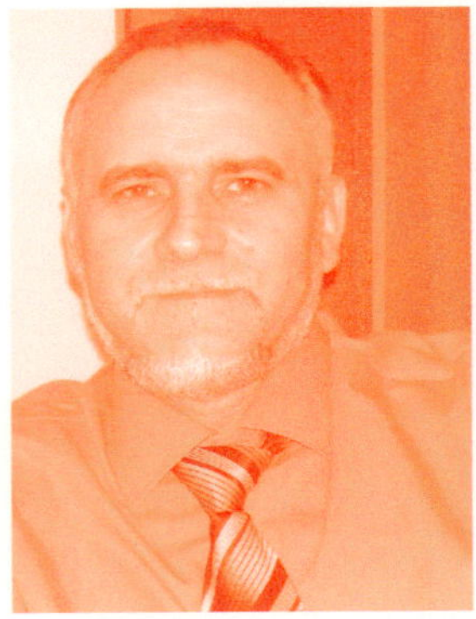
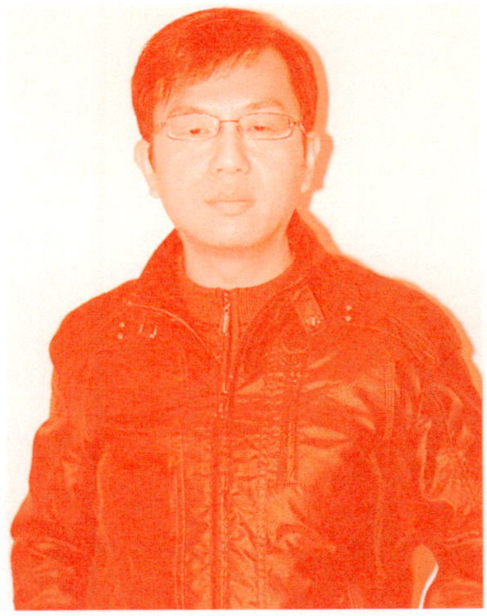
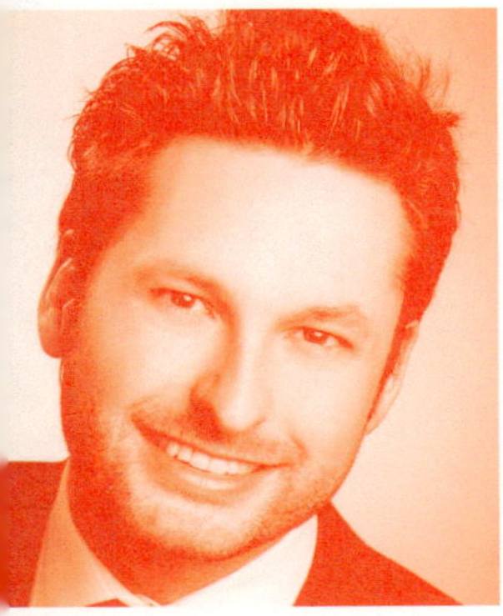
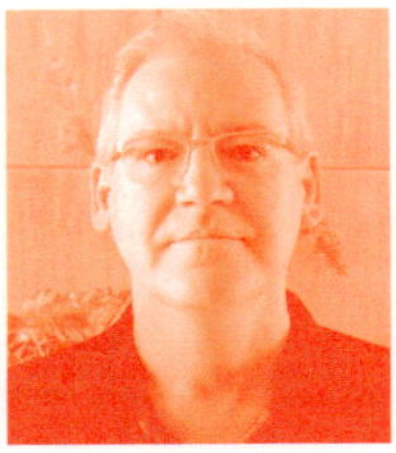

IntechOpen

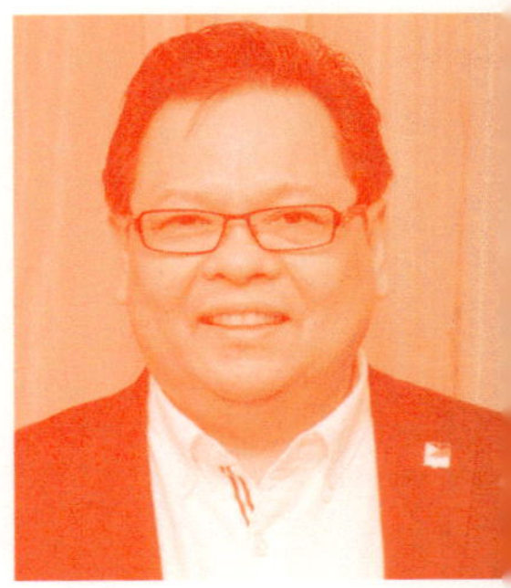
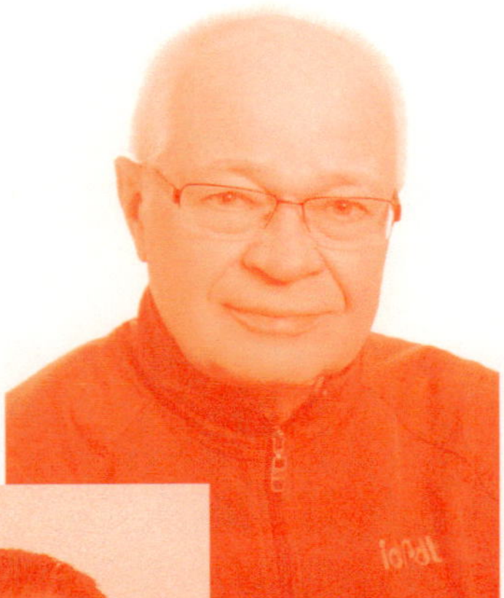
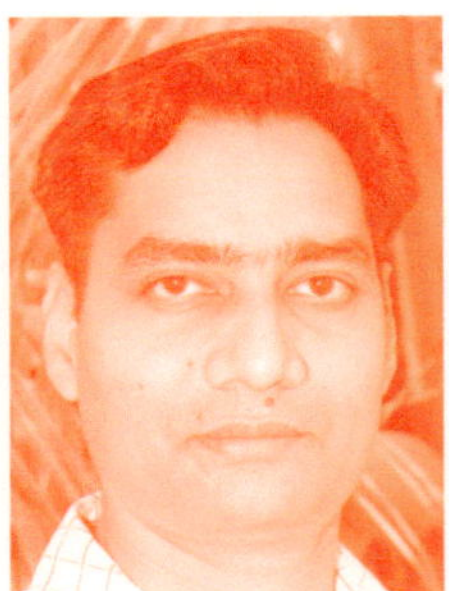
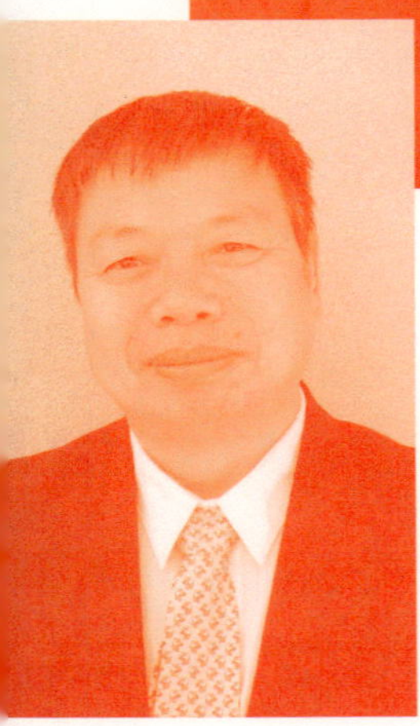
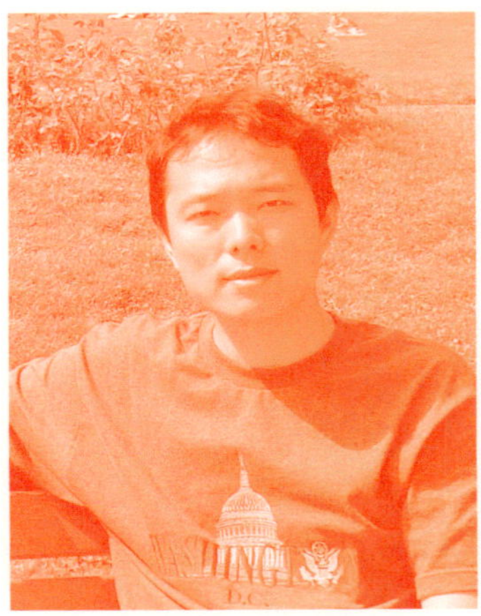
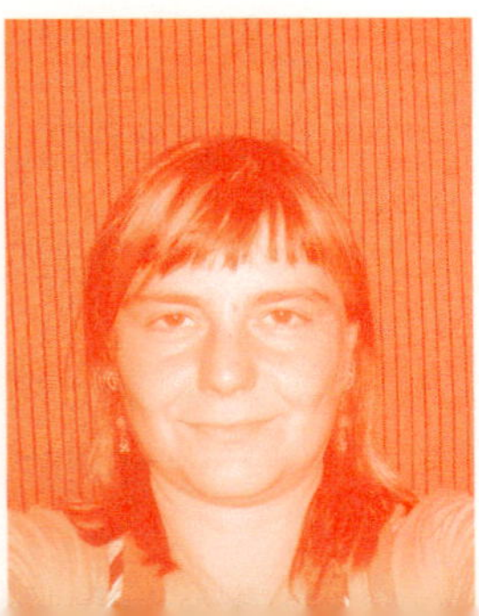

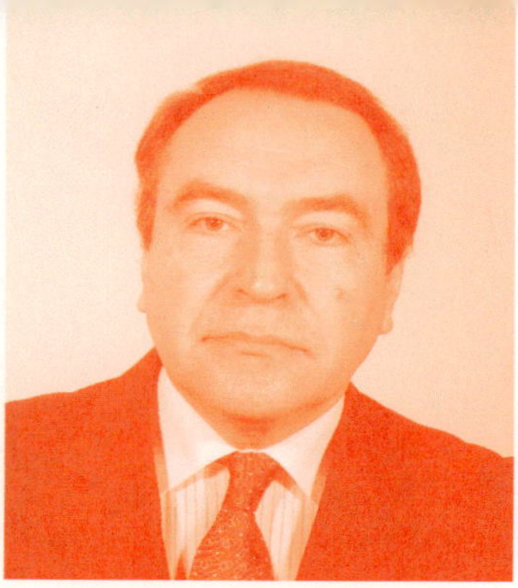
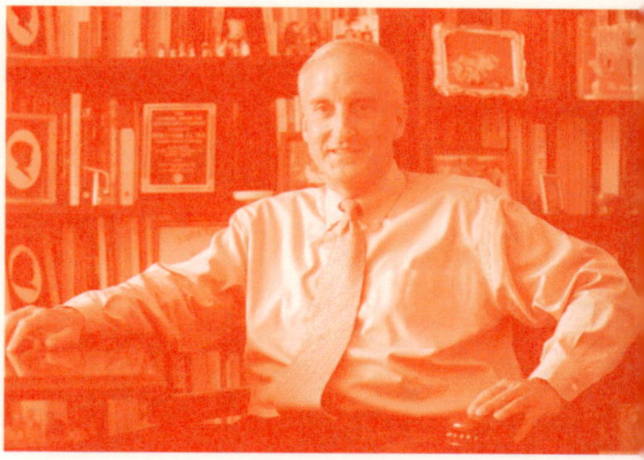
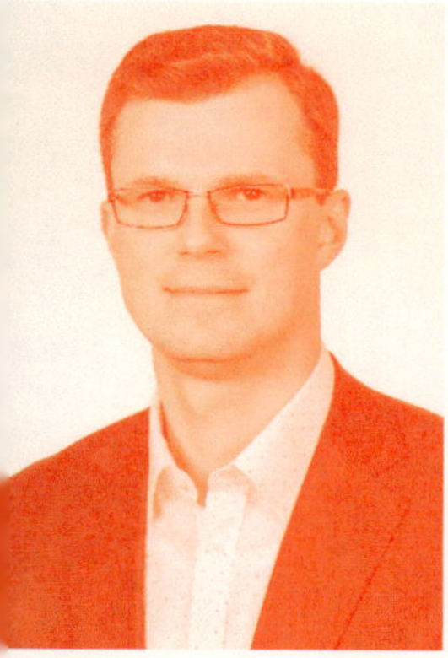
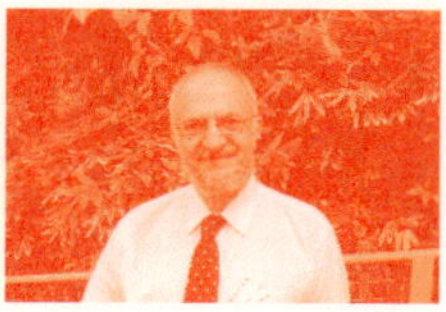
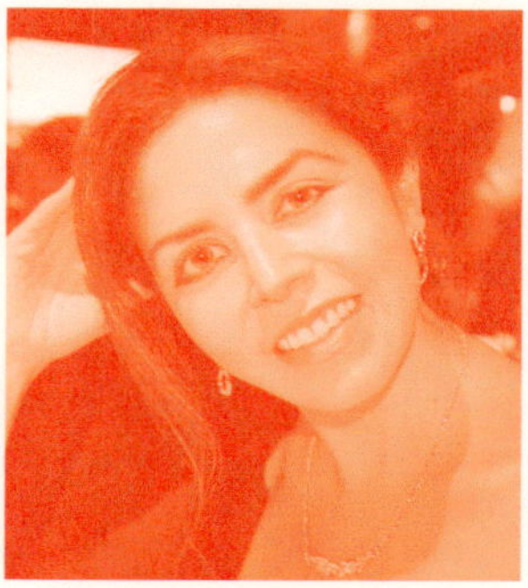

Supporting open minds since 2005

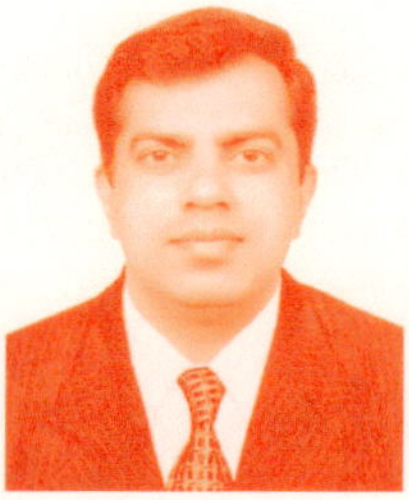
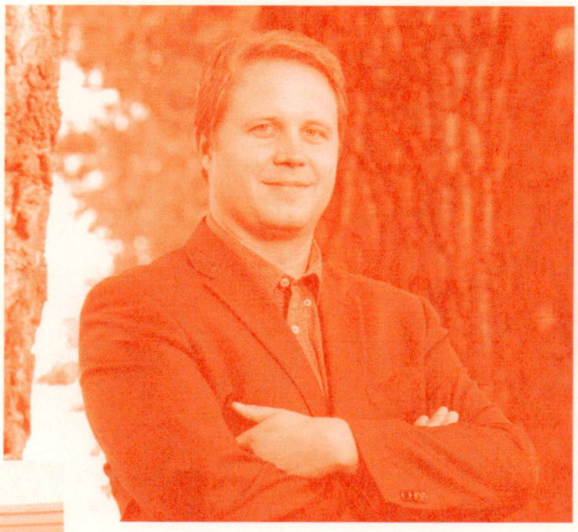
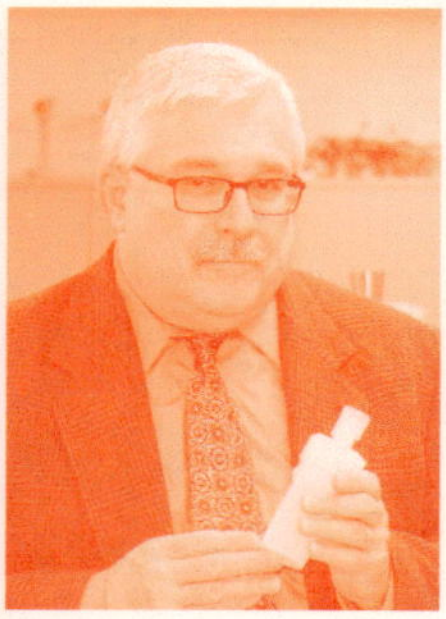
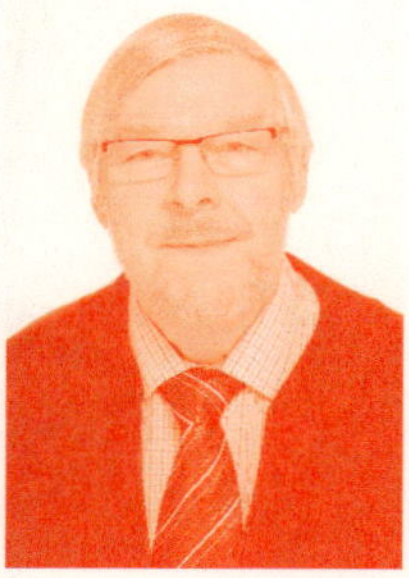
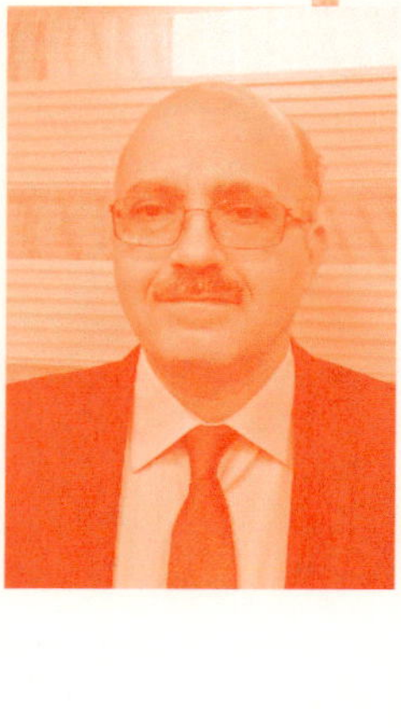
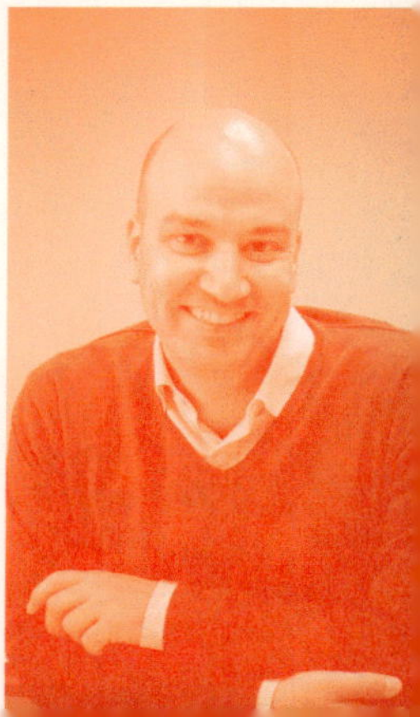
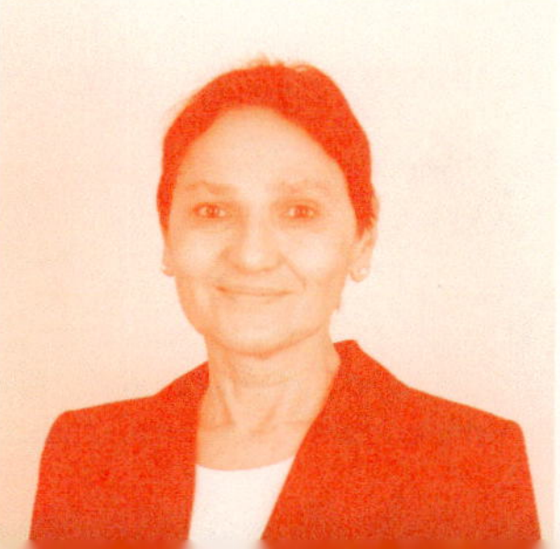

Recent Advances in Asthma Research and Treatments
http://dx.doi.org/10.5772/intechopen.91510
Edited by Svetlana P. Chapoval

Contributors
Callen Kwamboka Onyambu, Angeline Anyona Aywak, Sarah Kemunto Osiemo, Timothy Musila Mutala, Gulfidan Uzan, Utkarshani Jaimini, Amit Sheth, Xiaoyan Dong, Chao Wang, Yanhua Niu, Aşkın Gülsen, Svetlana P. Chapoval, Andrei I. Chapoval

First published in London, United Kingdom, 2022 by IntechOpen
IntechOpen is the global imprint of INTECHOPEN LIMITED, registered in England and Wales, registration number: 11086078, 5 Princes Gate Court, London, SW7 2QJ, United Kingdom
Printed in Croatia

British Library Cataloguing-in-Publication Data
A catalogue record for this book is available from the British Library

Additional hard and PDF copies can be obtained from orders@intechopen.com

Recent Advances in Asthma Research and Treatments
Edited by Svetlana P. Chapoval
p. cm.
Print ISBN 978-1-83969-205-5
Online ISBN 978-1-83969-206-2
eBook (PDF) ISBN 978-1-83969-207-9

For EU product safety concerns:
IN TECH d.o.o., Prolaz Marije Krucifikse Kozulić 3, 51000 Rijeka, Croatia, info@intechopen.com or visit our website at intechopen.com.

Meet the editor

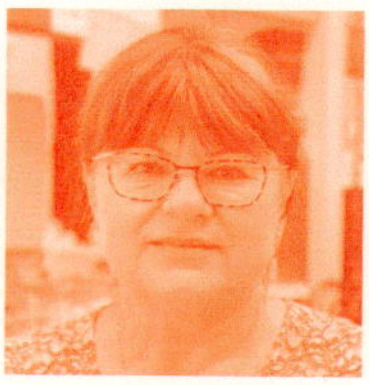

Svetlana Chapoval, MD, Ph.D., is an Assistant Professor of Microbiology and Immunology, Center for Vascular and Inflammatory Diseases, University of Maryland School of Medicine. She is a member of the Program in Oncology at the Greenebaum Comprehensive Cancer Center, Baltimore, Maryland. Dr. Chapoval obtained an MD from Pirogov Russian National Research Medical University and a Ph.D. from Gamaleya Scientific Research Institute of Epidemiology and Microbiology, Moscow, Russia. After her postdoctoral training in immunology at the Mayo Clinic and junior research faculty appointment in Pulmonary Medicine at Yale University, she joined the University of Maryland School of Medicine to continue her research on immunogenetics and immunoregulatory mechanisms of asthma pathophysiology. She established new research programs aimed at defining selected semaphorins as immune checkpoints and regulators of inflammation in immune-mediated diseases. Dr. Chapoval founded SemaPlex LLC to translate her research into preclinical development and clinical applications.

Contents

Preface **XI**

Chapter 1 **1**
Costimulation in Allergic Asthma: The Roles of B7 and Semaphorin Molecules
by Svetlana P. Chapoval and Andrei I. Chapoval

Chapter 2 **21**
Asthma and COVID-19
by Gulfidan Uzan

Chapter 3 **31**
Personalized Digital Phenotype Score, Healthcare Management and Intervention Strategies Using Knowledge Enabled Digital Health Framework for Pediatric Asthma
by Utkarshani Jaimini and Amit Sheth

Chapter 4 **45**
Epigenetic Regulation of Th2 Response in Asthma by Non-Coding RNAs
by Yanhua Niu, Chao Wang, Xiaoyan Dong and Nanbert Zhong

Chapter 5 **61**
Asthma Phenotypes and Current Biological Treatments
by Aşkın Gülşen

Chapter 6 **79**
Anaphylactic Reactions in Radiology Procedures
by Callen Kwamboka Onyambu, Angeline Anyona Aywak, Sarah Kemunto Osiemo and Timothy Musila Mutala

Preface

Asthma is a chronic lung disease characterized by episodes of airway narrowing and obstruction, causing wheezing, coughing, chest tightness, and shortness of breath [1]. The National Institute of Allergy and Infectious Disease (NIAID) in the United States specifies why asthma research is its priority. Asthma significantly reduces the quality of life. In addition to high medical expenses, asthma has substantial effects on work/school attendance and performance. Patients with asthma exacerbation often require emergency room visits and/or hospitalization. NIAID is especially committed to reducing the burden of this disease and its complications by supporting targeted research aimed at understanding asthma mechanisms, developing new prevention and treatment strategies, and understanding the involvement of environmental factors and human genetics in asthma initiation, progression, and severity.

Asthma triggers

Asthma is a Th2-driven systemic immunologic disease manifesting in lung pathology. Several factors bias the development of Th2 response to air pollution, traffic emissions, ozone, cigarette smoke, changes in the microbial environment, nutrition, and increased exposure to allergens [2]. NIAID supports research programs aimed at identifying the factors that contribute to asthma development and severity. It funds the Inner City Asthma Consortium (ICAC), a nationwide clinical network that conducts asthma research in nine US cities [3]. One of the studies from this Consortium determined the differences in clinical characteristics between easy-to-control and difficult-to-control asthma [4]. There was a relatively equal distribution of such asthma cases among the study participants, whereas around 22% of them fell into neither group. The study clearly points to allergen sensitizations as a major trigger of asthma exacerbations and the direct association of poorly controlled asthma with bronchodilator responsiveness, pulmonary physiology, rhinitis, and atopy. The more recent international study on the role of allergy in severe asthma by the Allergy and Asthma Severity EAACI Task Force was published in 2016 as a position document [4]. The document, in part, states that the proportion of severe asthma cases related to allergen exposure may be overestimated and other triggers such as fungal sensitization, smoking, and pollution contribute to severe asthma and must be considered during disease evaluation in patients.

The discussion by the international research expert group at the World Health Organization (WHO) meeting on the respiratory syncytial virus (RSV) and asthma was published in the journal Vaccine [5]. The main conclusions of the article are: (a) the casual association between lower respiratory tract infection with RSV and recurrent wheeze of early childhood in asthma is not fully established and requires further investigations; (b) there is no sufficient evidence that RSV monoclonal antibodies (mAbs) and potential future RSV vaccines will have a significant effect on asthma outcomes; and (c) there is a substantial public health threat from a severe acute RSV disease in young children, which requires the development of good clinical practice guidelines.

During the recent COVID-19 pandemic, taking into account that the SARS-CoV-2 virus primarily affects the respiratory system, reasonable concern was generated among health professionals on the viral effect on asthma patients, especially disease severity and exacerbation. One of the chapters in this book provides relevant information on this topic [6]. According to the International Primary Care Respiratory Group (IPCRG), which consists of 78 experts from 43 countries, patients are still struggling to differentiate their symptoms between asthma flare-ups and COVID-19 and might delay seeking care for either condition [7]. The IPCRG supports previous multiple observations concluding that asthma is not a risk factor for severe COVID-19, but patients taking oral corticosteroids may be at greater risk of severe COVID-19. The IPCRG recommendations include the use of protective equipment, lung function testing procedures, long-term use of oral steroids, and the application of biologics.

Asthma phenotypes and biologics

Asthma is widely recognized as heterogeneous inflammatory lung disease. One of the chapters in this book is dedicated to asthma phenotypes and biologics [8]. It focuses on high and low Th2 endotypes and provides a detailed overview of current biologics, their safety, and effectiveness.

The recently published article by Conrad and associates [9] details the clinical characteristics of asthma clusters in adults and in children. The article also provides an approach to asthma diagnosis and management in children where a healthcare provider defines asthma severity and control according to the National Heart, Lung, and Blood Institute (NHLBI) guidelines based on symptom frequency and medication use. The presence of comorbidities and the results of pulmonary function tests are also incorporated into this systemic approach, which can be used in any given patient.

Another asthma classification proposed by the multi-institutional research team supported by the NHLBI's Severe Asthma Research Program is based on imaging cluster analysis and its association with known clinical parameters [10]. To identify the patient's clinical clusters, the authors developed lung tissue imaging-based clusters using multiple variables that reflect the airway and parenchymal pathologies. The observed structural and functional alterations were associated with the pathophysiology of asthma, which provided a meaningful association of airway structural pathologies with clinical metrics. Asthma clustering can be used as a basis for the development of novel and efficient immunotherapeutic measures to fight the disease.

Tay and Foster [11] defined four asthma groups based on the cellular composition of lung inflammatory infiltrates: (1) eosinophilic (T2), (2) neutrophilic (T1), (3) mixed eosinophilic/ neutrophilic, and (4) paucigranulocytic. The authors state that current treatments for asthma are non-specific and not often effective; therefore, there is a great need for the development and application of novel therapies. The wide range of new-generation biologics showed promising results as effective treatments for severe asthma. Those biologics specifically target the critical molecules of the Th2 immune response such as IgE, IL-4, IL-5, and IL-13. The authors also admit that biologics for non-Th2 asthma are difficult to develop and assess, as it is unclear what drives such asthma. Nevertheless, a chapter by Dr. Aşkın Gülşen [8] discusses IL-17-, IL-9-, TSLP-, and PGD2-directed therapies and their potential in the treatment of eosinophilic and non-eosinophilic asthma.

Selected B7 and semaphorin molecules might provide new targets for biologics or serve as new biologics (reviewed in [12]). Another chapter in this book summarizes current knowledge concerning the roles of B7 family immunomodulatory ligands in asthma and analyzes the potential functions of emerging new B7-H4, B7-H5, and B7-H7 molecules. It also provides insight into the roles of neuroimmune semaphorins in allergy and asthma. The discussed data will help to design more specific and efficient novel therapies to fight these diseases, which represent a significant public health burden.

Several research groups examined the roles of selected miRNAs, lncRNAs, and circRNAs in Th2-mediated inflammation in asthma (reviewed [13]). Another chapter summarizes the most significant advances in RNA research over the past years focused on miRNA-19a, -106a, -145, -146a, -155, -214, and others. The chapter discusses the regulation of a Th1/Th2 balance by several lncRNAs such as MALTA1, LNC_000127, PVT1, and others. The mechanistic interplay between miRNAs and lncRNAs and the effect of circRNAs on Th2 response in asthma showed that all studied RNAs play important regulatory roles in disease and need to be evaluated further as potential druggable targets for therapeutic intervention.

Several mobile applications are currently available for monitoring and collecting patient data [14, 15]. One such advanced application useful for physicians and patients, kHealth: Knowledge-enabled Digital Healthcare Framework, is reported in this book [16]. This mobile app is aimed at monitoring and managing asthma symptoms, medication adherence, lung function, daily activity, sleep quality, and indoor and outdoor environmental triggers. Physicians can use kHealth technology for both in-person and telemedicine appointments and patients can use it to monitor, evaluate, and manage their asthma symptoms and treatments continuously.

Summary

There have been many advances in our understanding of asthma genetics and immunologic mechanisms over the past several decades. Many scientific advances have been made in defining the distinct asthma phenotypes, which require personalized treatment strategies with available therapeutics. The identification of novel biologics can potentially lead to the development of better therapeutics. This book discusses some of these novel findings.

Svetlana P. Chapoval, MD, Ph.D.
Assistant Professor,
Department of Microbiology and Immunology,
Center for Vascular and Inflammatory Diseases,
University of Maryland School of Medicine,
Baltimore, Maryland, USA

Founder, SemaPlex LLC,
Ellicott City, Maryland, USA

References

[1] https://www.niaid.nih.gov/diseases-conditions/asthma

[2] Chapoval SP, David CS. Identification of antigenic epitopes on human allergens: studies with HLA transgenic mice. Environ Health Perspect. 2003 Feb;111(2):245-50.

[3] https://www.niaid.nih.gov/news-events/niaid-sponsored-study-finds-factors-influence-asthma-severity-inner-city-children

[4] Pongracic JA, Krouse RZ, Babineau DC, Zoratti EM, Cohen RT, Wood RA, Khurana Hershey GK, Kercsmar CM, Gruchalla RS, Kattan M, Teach SJ, Johnson CC, Bacharier LB, Gern JE, Sigelman SM, Gergen PJ, Togias A, Visness CM, Busse WW, Liu AH. Distinguishing characteristics of difficult-to-control asthma in inner-city children and adolescents. J Allergy Clin Immunol. 2016 Oct;138(4):1030-1041.

[5] Driscoll AJ, Arshad SH, Bont L, Brunwasser SM, Cherian T, Englund JA,et al. Does respiratory syncytial virus lower respiratory illness in early life cause recurrent wheeze of early childhood and asthma? Critical review of the evidence and guidance for future studies from a World Health Organization-sponsored meeting. Vaccine. 2020 Mar 4;38(11):2435-2448.

[6] Uzan G. Asthma and COVID-19. In: P. DS, editor. Recent Advances in Asthma Research and Treatments [Working Title] [Internet]. London: IntechOpen; 2021 [cited 2022 Feb 15]. Available from: https://www.intechopen.com/online-first/75230 doi: 10.5772/intechopen.96211

[7] Bousquet J, Jutel M, Akdis CA, Klimek L, Pfaar O, Nadeau KC, et al. ARIA-EAACI statement on asthma and COVID-19 (June 2, 2020). Allergy. 2021 Mar;76(3):689-697.

[8] Gülşen A. Asthma Phenotypes and Current Biological Treatments. In: P. DS, editor. Recent Advances in Asthma Research and Treatments [Working Title] [Internet]. London: IntechOpen; 2021 [cited 2022 Feb 15]. Available from: https://www.intechopen.com/online-first/76328 doi: 10.5772/intechopen.97376

[9] Conrad LA, Cabana MD, Rastogi D. Defining pediatric asthma: phenotypes to endotypes and beyond. Pediatr Res. 2020 Nov 10:10.1038/s41390-020-01231-6

[10] Choi S, Hoffman EA, Wenzel SE, Castro M, Fain S, Jarjour N, Schiebler ML, Chen K, Lin CL; National Heart, Lung and Blood Institute's Severe Asthma Research Program. Quantitative computed tomographic imaging-based clustering differentiates asthmatic subgroups with distinctive clinical phenotypes. J Allergy Clin Immunol. 2017 Sep;140(3):690-700.e8.

[11] Tay HL, Foster PS. Biologics or immunotherapeutics for asthma? Pharmacol Res. 2020 Aug;158:104782.

[12] Chapoval SP, Chapoval AI. Costimulation in Allergic Asthma: The Roles of B7 and Semaphorin Molecules. In: P. DS, editor. Recent Advances in Asthma Research and Treatments [Working Title] [Internet]. London: IntechOpen; 2022 [cited 2022 Feb 15]. Available from: https://www.intechopen.com/online-first/80428 doi: 10.5772/intechopen.102631

[13] Niu Y, Wang C, Dong X, Zhong N. Epigenetic Regulation of Th2 Response in Asthma by Non-Coding RNAs. In: P. DS, editor. Recent Advances in Asthma Research and Treatments

[Working Title] [Internet]. London: IntechOpen; 2021 [cited 2022 Feb 15]. Available from: https://www.intechopen.com/online-first/76303 doi: 10.5772/intechopen.97328

[14] Himes BE, Leszinsky L, Walsh R, Hepner H, Wu AC. Mobile Health and Inhaler-Based Monitoring Devices for Asthma Management. J Allergy Clin Immunol Pract. 2019 Nov-Dec;7(8):2535-2543.

[15] Sleurs K, Seys SF, Bousquet J, Fokkens WJ, Gorris S, Pugin B, Hellings PW. Mobile health tools for the management of chronic respiratory diseases. Allergy. 2019 Jul;74(7):1292-1306.

[16] Jaimini U, Sheth A. Personalized Digital Phenotype Score, Healthcare Management and Intervention Strategies using Knowledge Enabled Digital Health Framework for Pediatric Asthma. In: P. DS, editor. Recent Advances in Asthma Research and Treatments [Working Title] [Internet]. London: IntechOpen; 2021 [cited 2022 Feb 15]. Available from: https://www.intechopen.com/online-first/76503 doi: 10.5772/intechopen.97430

Chapter 1

Costimulation in Allergic Asthma: The Roles of B7 and Semaphorin Molecules

Svetlana P. Chapoval and Andrei I. Chapoval

Abstract

It is well established that allergic asthma is T cell-driven disease where CD4+ T cells of Th2 phenotype play a critical role in disease initiation and maintenance. There are several critical steps in the induction of Th2 type immune response to the allergen. The first critical step is the antigen processing and presentation of allergen-derived peptides in the context of specific major histocompatibility Class II (MHCII) molecules by antigen-presenting cells (APC). Recognition of this complex by T cell receptor (TCR) and interaction of costimulatory ligands with corresponding receptors represents the second step in T cell activation. As the third part of optimal T cell differentiation, proliferation, and expansion, several cytokines, integrins, and chemokines get involved in the fine-tuning of DC-T cell interaction and activation. Multiple recent evidences point to the selected members of B7 and semaphorin families as important checkpoints providing a fine-tuning regulation of immune response. In this book chapter, we discuss the properties of costimulatory molecules and address their roles in allergic asthma.

Keywords: asthma, immune response, costimulation, immune checkpoints, B7 family molecules, semaphorins

1. Introduction

Allergic asthma is a Th2-driven, immunological chronic disease [1]. CD4+ T cells of Th2 phenotype secreting Th2 cytokines such as IL-4, IL-5, and IL-13 play a critical role in asthma initiation and propagation [2]. In this book chapter, we address the question of how different costimulatory molecules influence the allergic immune response which is central to asthma pathogenesis.

The initial step in the immune response is the antigen capture and processing by APC. APC subdivide into "professional" such as dendritic cells (DC), B cells, and macrophages, and "unprofessional" such as epithelial cells, fibroblasts, basophils, eosinophils, ILC2 (type 2 innate lymphoid cells), which normally have other functions in tissues and do not act as APC [3–5]. Antigenic epitopes derived from a captured allergen are presented to T cells in the context of specific MHC (human leukocyte antigen, HLA, for human cells) molecules [1]. This is the first signal for T cell activation, whereas a second signal is derived from costimulation where specific costimulatory molecules on APC interact with their receptors on T cells (**Figure 1**) [6]. The first

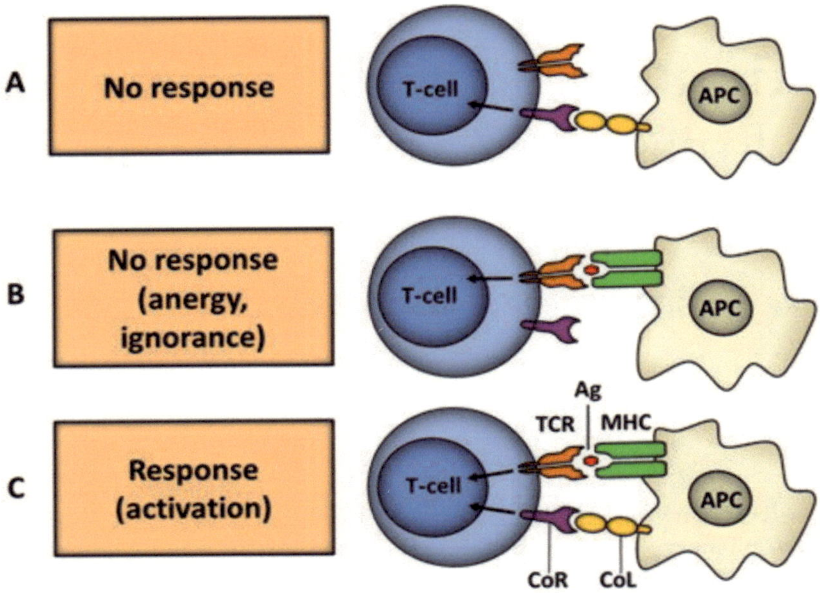

Figure 1.
The two-signal model of the T-cell activation. (a) Functions of the immune checkpoint molecules (IChMs) are completely dependent on the first signal because the interaction of the receptor (Co-R) on T-cells with the ligand (Co-L) on APCs (the second signal) do not result in an activation of T-cells without the first signal. (b) T-cell activation has not occurred in the absence of the second signal. In several cases, the absence of the second signal leads to T-cell tolerance and anergy. (c) the correct activation of T-lymphocytes occurs after the TCR interaction with the MHC-presented peptide (Ag) (the first signal) and after the interaction of a ligand of the B7 family (Co-L) with its receptor (Co-R) (the second signal). A synergism of the two signals results in an optimal activation of T-cells.

signal alone does not lead to the immune response to allergen (**Figure 1**), it rather induces T cell unresponsiveness or "anergy" [6, 7].

The members of the B7 family are the most characterized immunomodulatory ligands that bind to receptors on lymphocytes. They can act as costimulators or inhibitors/checkpoints. Currently, there are eleven known representatives of the B7 family, namely: B7–1 (CD80), B7–2 (CD86), B7-H1 (PD-L1, CD274), B7-DC (PDCD1LG2, PD-L2, CD273), B7-H2 (B7RP1, ICOS-L, CD275), B7-H3 (CD276), B7-H4 (B7x, B7S1, Vtcn1), B7-H5 (VISTA, Platelet receptor Gi24, SISP1), B7-H6 (NCR3LG1), B7-H7 (HHLA2), and ILDR2 (the synonyms of IChM names of the B7 family are given in parentheses) [7, 8]. Two molecules of B7 family proteins [9], B7–1 and B7–2, are the best characterized costimulators [7, 8]. Their ligation of CD28 expressed on T cells leads to T cell activation whereas interaction with cytotoxic T lymphocyte-associated antigen 4 (CTLA-4) functions as an inhibitory signal.

Multiple recent reports pointed to selected semaphorin family [10, 11] members acting as checkpoints in the immune response regulating optimal T cell activation and cytokine production [10, 12]. Semaphorins alone are unable to induce or suppress T cell activation regulated by a combination of signals 1 and 2 but can significantly potentiate or downregulate it [10, 12]. Moreover, their involvement in asthmatic disease development has been supported by several recent publications (reviewed in [13–15] establishing them as potential immunomodulatory targets.

The goal of this book chapter is to discuss the roles of these molecules in asthma and provide the ground for their therapeutic use in disease prevention, management, or treatment.

2. B7 family members in asthma

2.1 B7: 1 and B7: 2

Asthma is Th2 cell-driven disease with Th2 type cytokines such as IL-4, IL-5, and IL-13 driving the disease pathology [2]. The effect of costimulation in asthma has been a subject of several decades' of research. The differential role of two B7 family members in allergic response has been extensively studied and described in multiple articles published in the late 1990-s (16–19, reviewed in 20, 21). The work by Freeman et al. [16] questioned the functional necessity of two known at that time B7 family members. Using the *in vitro* cell cultures and distinct transfectants, they reported that both B7–1 and B7–2 effectively and equally costimulate T cells to produce IL-2 and IFNγ, however, B7–2 was more efficient in costimulation of IL-4 production with cell priming and especially with a repetitive cell stimulation, whereas B7–1 was efficient for GM-CSF production. Similarly, anti-B7–2 mAb significantly reduced the induction of IL-4 mRNA in a primary human allogeneic MLR whereas anti-B7–1 mAb failed to do so. The work by Van Neerven [17] addressed the same question as the discussed above research but in different experimental settings, namely the stimulation of human PBMC obtained from allergic and non-allergic persons *in vitro* with house dust mite allergen (HDM) in the presence or absence of B7–1 or B7–2 blocking Abs, or CTLA-Ig. CTLA4-Ig was efficient in inhibiting allergen-induced cell proliferation and cytokine production. The proliferation of CTLA4-Ig-treated cells was partially restored by stimulating them with anti-CD28 mAb which indicated that CTLA4-Ig inhibits the interaction of CD28 with both, CD80 and CD86. Interestingly, anti-CD86 mAb inhibited the HDM-induced cell proliferation similarly to CTLA4-Ig but with less degree of inhibition. However, the addition of anti-CD80 blocking mAb to the anti- CD86 mAb treated cells resulted in identical inhibition as with CTLA4-Ig. This report suggested that the costimulation inactivation could be efficient in the downregulation of allergen-dependent Th2 responses in asthmatic patients (**Figure 2**). The research by Larche et al. [18] used allergen stimulation of human PBMC and cells obtained by alveolar lavages to examine B7–1 and B7–2 dependence of T cell immune response. While allergen-induced PBMC proliferation and cytokine production were inhibited by the use of CTLA4-Ig and anti-B7–2 Ab in cell cultures, anti-B7–1 Ab showed no effect. Moreover, HDM-induced broncho-alveolar lavage (BAL) T cell proliferation was also B7–2 but not B7–1 dependent. This study further supported the notion that T cell costimulation-targeted therapy could be beneficial in asthma management. The study by Jaffar et al. [19] stimulated with HDM allergen the explants from endobronchial mucosal biopsies obtained from asthmatic patients. Although this study did not address the requirement of individual B7–1 or B7–2 molecules in anti-allergic T cell response, it clearly demonstrated the requirement of B7/CD28 costimulation in IL-5 and IL-13 production using a novel tool for asthma research, the bronchial explant system. Moreover, they were the first to demonstrate a significant difference in cytokine profile in bronchial explants between asthmatic and non-asthmatic lungs.

2.2 B7-H1 (PD-L1) and B7-DC (PD-L2)

The B7 homolog 1 (B7-H1) shares the same inducible PD-1 receptor on T cells with B7-DC (reviewed in 20, 21). While B7-H1 is constitutively expressed on monocytes and is downregulated with cell activation, B7-DC expression is induced by cell activation (reviewed in 7, 8, 20). Functionally, it was speculated that PDL-1

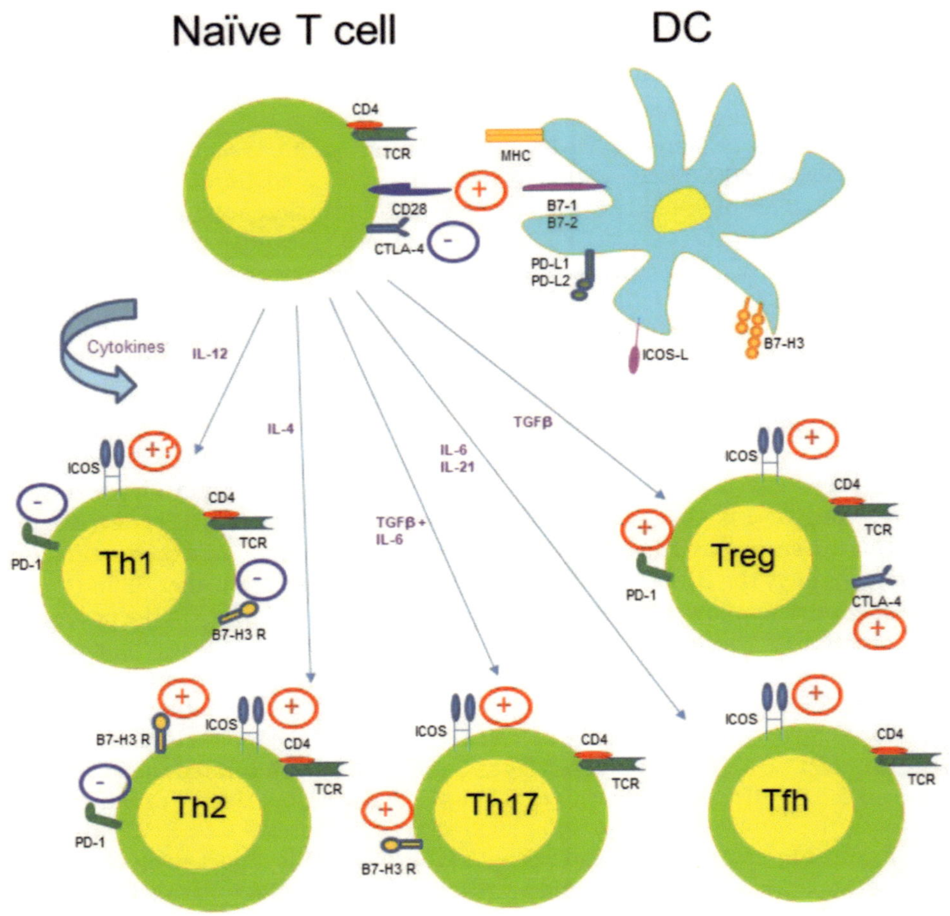

Figure 2.
Role of costimulation in T cell immune response and asthma. a. B7–1 and B7–2 interaction with CTLA-4 contributes to suppressive activity of allergen-specific Treg cells whereas their interaction with CD28 costimulates Th1 and Th2 responses. b. ICOS-L – ICOS interaction regulates Th2 effector cell function; it is efficient in stimulation of IL-4 and IL-10 production but not IFNγ. It regulates Th2 cell infiltration into lungs, promotes B cell differentiation and IgE production, contributes to AHR. This pathway also regulates IL-10 production in Treg cells. c. PD-L1 interaction with PD-1 receptor play a protective role in allergic asthma as it was reported to drive a differentiation of Treg cells and to downregulate contact hypersensitivity reaction. On the other hand, the use of neutralizing anti-PD-1 ab in vivo decreased eosinophilic lung infiltration but increased AHR and lung neutrophilia. d. PD-L2 interaction with PD-1 receptor downregulates allergic asthmatic response by suppressing Th2 cell activation, AHR, eosinophil infiltration, and IgE production. e. B7-H3 interaction with unknown receptor promotes Th2 and Th17 cell differentiation, lung infiltration by eosinophils, AHR, IL-4 and IL-17 production.

may suppress Th1-mediated inflammation and PDL-2 may suppress Th2-mediated inflammation (**Figure 2**) [20, 21]. The expression and regulation of PD-L1 and PD-L2 in asthma were analyzed using a segmental challenge of human lungs with allergen followed by BAL [22]. This study was initiated to clarify the importance of these costimulators in human asthma as previous reports using mouse models of the disease gave conflicting results [23–25]. The mouse lung expression levels of PD-L1 and PD-L2 were significantly upregulated by the OVA challenge [25]. However, the treatment of DC with CPG DNA, CD40L, GM-CSF, LPS, and IFN-γ led to the increased expression of PD-L2 on the cell surface whereas IL-4 and IL-13 induced the highest PD-L2 expression on DC among all mentioned above stimuli [25]. Interestingly, Th2 cytokines induce PD-L2 expression on DC but not B7–1 or B7–2 expression suggesting a regulatory role of this costimulatory in Th2 cell activation. *In vivo* treatment of mice with recombinant PD-L2-Fc resulted in a Th2-like inflammation in murine lungs. Such effect of PD-L2-Fc could be explained by a potential PD-L2-Fc blocking of the inhibitory interaction of cell-associated PD-L2 or PD-L1 with PD-1 or by a potential PD-L2-Fc interaction with a second receptor and enhancement of T cell activation via a PD-1-independent mechanism. This alternative yet unidentified receptor may dominate the inhibitory PD-1 receptor *in vivo*. The observed negative correlation between PD-1 expression by circulating CD4+ T cells and IgE concentrations in serum in asthma patients suggested a protective role of PD-L1 in allergic asthma [22]. However, there was an increase in blood and a decrease in BAL of PD-1+ CD4+ T cells after segmental bronchial challenge with the allergen [22]. The authors concluded that the up-regulation of PD-L1 and downregulation of PD-L2 on endobronchial DC subsets favor a Th2 inflammation in their human asthma model based on a segmental lung allergen challenge. They propose that modulating PD-1 ligand-mediated pathways by blocking PD-L1 or activating PD-L2 signaling could be a promising immunomodulatory approach in allergic asthma management. A more recent study has shown that in the *in vivo* experimental model of HDM-induced asthma anti-PD-L1 mAb completely abrogated eosinophil recruitment and PD-1/PD-L1 blockade by the use of neutralizing mAb to either PD-1 or PD-L1 led to the enhanced airway hyperreactivity (AHR) due to activation of Th17 cells and resulting increase of airway neutrophilia [26]. The authors identified the increased frequency of CD4 + IFNγ + and CD4 + IL-17A+ cells in PD-1-deficient (Pdcd1−/−) mice which directly correlated with higher levels of circulating IFNγ and IL-17A. This study goes in accord with previous research establishing allergic asthma as a mix Th2/Th17 response. Clinical observation in patients with chronic occupational asthma showed a persistent PD-L2 expressing mDC-mediated Th2 response that was partially PD-L2-dependent [27]. This suggests that other costimulators participate in Th2 activation in the asthmatic setting.

2.3 B7-H2 and ICOS

Another pair of the B7 family ligand and its receptor involved in the regulation of T cell activation comprises of B7-H2 and ICOS (Inducible CO-Stimulator) (**Figure 2**). It was originally shown that the engagement of ICOS by B7-H2 on CD4+ T cells increased the production of Th1 (IFN-γ and TNFα) and Th2 (IL-4, IL-5, and IL-10) cytokines [28–30]. ICOS-deficient mice were unable to induce the allergen-specific IgE responses when compared to WT mice which demonstrated an important role of ICOS:B7-H2 interaction in the induction of IgE production [31]. It was shown recently that the injection of anti-B7-H2 mAb resulted in the reduction of inflammation and Th2 cytokines production in the mouse model of allergic asthma [32]. Moreover, blocking the ICOS:B7-H2 interaction on human ILC2s reduced AHR and lung inflammation in the experimental asthma model [33]. In addition, it was demonstrated that in contrast to wild-type counterparts, B7-H2 deficient mice did not develop AHR after OVA sensitization and challenge [34].

2.4 B7-H3 and other B7-H molecules

To investigate the contribution of B7-H3 to the development of allergic asthma, mice were treated with antiB7-H3 blocking Ab during the course of OVA sensitization and challenges [35]. Anti-B7-H3 mAb treatment of mice at the experimental asthma induction phase (days 7–18 after allergen priming) suppressed allergic lung inflammation including eosinophilic infiltration, airway mucus hypersecretion, downregulated the number of B7-H3+ cells in the lung tissues as compared with the immunoglobulin G (IgG) treated control group. In addition, anti-B7-H3 mAb inhibited IL-4 and IL-17 levels and increased the expression IFN-γ in BALF of allergen-treated mice. However, anti-B7-H3 mAb treatment did not show an inhibitory effect on any measured asthma parameters at the effector phase (days 21–27 after priming). Nevertheless, B7-H3 blockage can provide a novel therapeutic approach for allergic asthma especially if used in a combination with immunotherapies that work in the effector phase. Two years later the same group of scientists reported an association of asthma exacerbation with increased levels of B7-H3 expression in the peripheral blood of asthmatic children which was significantly decreased by the use of steroids [36]. Their further studies in an animal model of asthma showed that recombinant B7-H3 administration to the mouse lungs in the time-frame of allergen priming (days 0 to 14), but before challenge (days 21, 27), significantly upregulate all parameters of allergic response such as inflammatory cell infiltration to the lung tissues, Th1 and Th2 cytokine levels in BAL and plasma, allergen-specific IgE production, and Th2/Th17 cell proliferation and cytokine levels [37].

The roles of other B7 family members such as B7-H4, B7-H5, and B7-H7 in asthma have never been investigated. Conflicting data on B7-H7 costimulation results led to a proposed concept of dual functionality as it is in the case of B7–1/B7–2 and CD28/CTLA-4. As an example, B7-H7 receptor CD28H could serve as an immunostimulatory receptor for T cell activation whereas KIR3DL3 could inhibit immune responses upon ligation of B7-H7 [38]. On the other hand, CD28H which is a CD28 homolog absent in mice but present in human serves as a functional receptor for B7-H5 [39]. B7-H5/CD28H interaction selectively costimulates human T-cell growth and cytokine production via an AKT-dependent signaling cascade. Interestingly, CD28H is constitutively expressed on all naïve T cells and its expression decreased with cell activation and is lost on terminally differentiated effector CD45RA + CCR7 – T cells [39]. Basically, the effector cytokine-producing CD4+ T helper cells and FoxP3+ CD4+ T reg cells lack CD28H expression. The authors associate such loss of expression for effector cells with repetitive cell stimulation. Moreover, the pattern on B7-H5 expression in peripheral tissue suggests that B7-H5/CD28H interaction is critical for the co-stimulation of newly generated effector or effector/memory T cells at the periphery. B7-H6 was not detected in normal human tissues but was expressed on human tumor cells [40]. B7-H6 triggers NKp30-mediated activation of human NK cells [40]. In summary, the roles of B7-H4, B7-H5, B7-H6, and B7-H7 in allergic asthma are long overdue to be determined.

2.5 ILDR2 in the immune response

Ildr2 (Ig-like domain-containing receptor 2), the gene encoding the murine ortholog (formerly designated "Lisch-like") was originally identified as a modifier of susceptibility to type 2 diabetes in obese mice [41]. Its expression level was associated with reduced β- cell number and reproduction and with persistent mild hypoinsulinemic hyperglycemia [41]. A new immunomodulatory function of this B7-like homolog protein has been recently reported by Hecht and associates [42]. They showed that the administration of a recombinant ILDR2-mFc protein to mice displayed a therapeutic effect in a model of rheumatoid arthritis. It induced an increase in the IgG1/IgG2a ratio which suggested a shift from the proinflammatory pro-rheumatic Th1 responses to anti-inflammatory Th2 responses. The ILDR2 upregulation was reported previously for DC cultures when they were stimulated to become DC2-like cell that promotes Th2 response [43]. Therefore, ILDR2 has a promoting effect on allergic diseases, however, it has never been investigated directly.

3. Neuroimmune semaphorins in asthma

Several neuronal guidance proteins, known as semaphorin molecules, function in the immune system. This dual tissue performance has led to them being defined as "neuroimmune semaphorins" [44]. They have been shown to regulate T cell activation by serving as immune checkpoints (**Figure 3**) [12]. Neuroimmune semaphorins are either constitutively or inducibly expressed on immune cells. The T cell co-stimulatory action of neuroimmune semaphorins requires the presence of two signals: signal one provided by TCR/MHC engagement and signal two arises from B7/CD28 interaction. Thus, neuroimmune semaphorins serve as a "signal three" for immune cell activation by supporting their polarization, expansion, differentiation, and regulating the intensity of immune response. This book chapter summarizes the current knowledge on the structure and receptors for several neuroimmune semaphorins involved in the immune response and their role in allergic asthma.

3.1 Sema3A and Sema3E

Sema3A, previously known as chick collapsin 1, SemD, or Sema III, was discovered in the 1990s. In the nervous system, it functions either as a repulsive agent for axonal outgrowth or an attractive agent for apical dendrite growth [45–48]. Sema3A is a glycoprotein with an Ig-like C2-type domain, a PSI (cysteine-rich module in extracellular portion) domain, and a Sema domain. Antipenko and associates [49] reported the crystal structure of Sema3A and identified a neuropilin (NRP) binding site and a potential plexin interaction site. Further studies demonstrated the physiologic receptors for Sema3A which consist of NRP/Plexin complexes where NRP1 serves as a ligand-binding receptor whereas Plexin A1 functions as a signaling receptor [50, 51]. The secreted 95 kDa forms of Sema3A can further undergo a proteolytic cleavage forming the 65 kDa forms [49], which have decreased activity toward neurons [52, 53]. The cryoEM of extracellular complex of Sema3A, PlexinA4, and NRP1 at 3.7 Å resolution demonstrated a large symmetric 2:2:2 molecular assembly in which each subunit makes multiple interactions with others [54].

The immunomodulatory role of Sema3A in allergic asthma has been extensively studied by the laboratory of Dr. Vadasz at Technion, Israel [55–57]. When examining the serum levels of Sema3A in asthmatic patients with different stages of disease severity they have determined that Sema3A was significantly downregulated in both severe and moderate asthmatic patients when compared to that of healthy individuals [55]. Low levels of Sema3A correlated with asthma severity. Purified CD4 + T cells from asthmatic patients were incubated with recombinant human (rh) Sema3A protein for 24 h what led to a higher number of Treg cells as compared to similarly conditioned cell cultures from healthy controls [55]. Moreover, rhSema3A affected Treg cells directly by inducing a higher Foxp3 expression. Considering the results of these clinical studies and established downregulatory role of Treg cells in asthma, it is logical to conclude that Sema3A plays an inhibitory role in allergic disease in part by inducing and stabilizing Treg cells. Indeed, the low expression of Sema3A was noticed in the nasal epithelium in the animal model of allergic rhinitis as compared to control mice [58]. Re-introduction of recombinant Sema3A to the mouse nose alleviated sneezing and nasal rubbing symptoms in allergic mice. When rhSema3A was administered intraperitoneally to the mice treated with allergen, a downregulation of lung inflammatory response and angiogenesis was observed [56, 57]. However, the full understanding of the mechanisms of lung inflammation and angiogenesis suppression by Sema3A is still ill-defined.

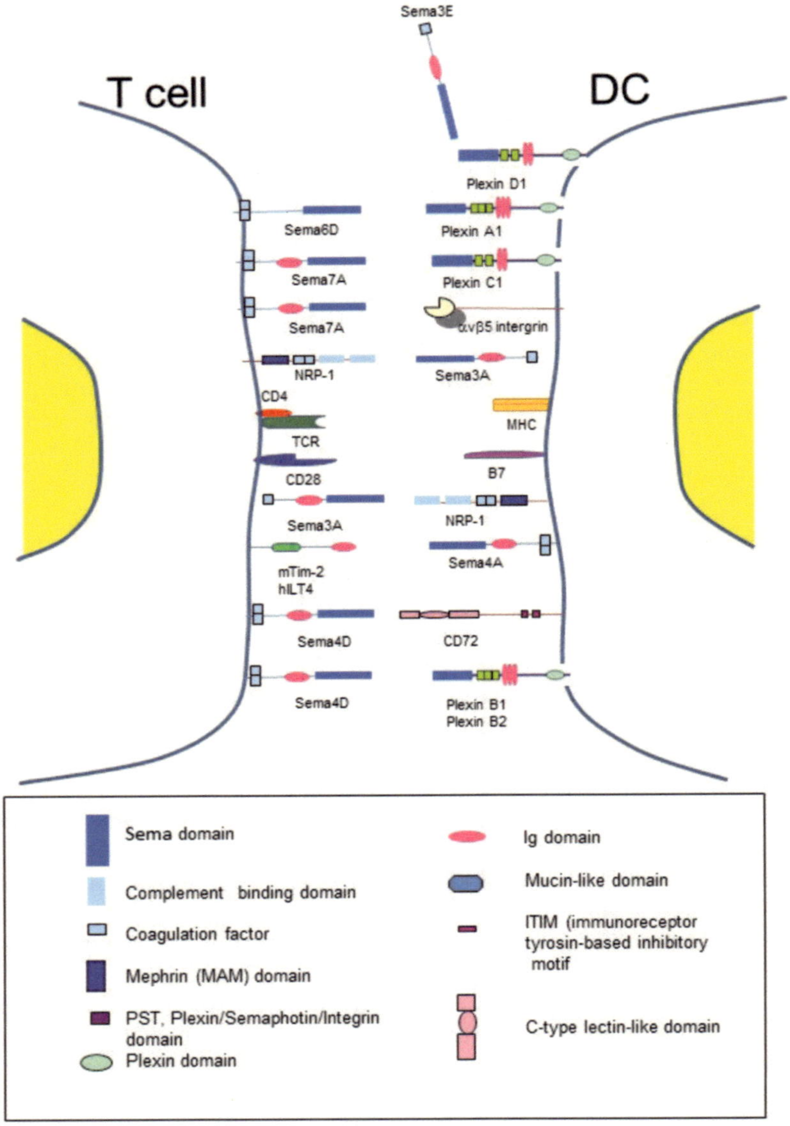

Figure 3.
Neuroimmune semaphorins in T cell – DC crosstalk. a. Sema3A. Sema3A inhibits T cell activation. Low constitutive levels of Sema3A on DC are upregulated with cell activation. DC surface-expressed and soluble Sema3A inhibit T cell proliferation presumably acting through NRP-1. Sema3A inhibits DC activation and chemotaxis. Inducible T cell-expressed and soluble Sema3A use NRP-1 and NRP-2 as ligand-binding receptors and NRP-associated Plexin A1 and A2 as signaling receptors to regulate DC activation and chemotaxis. b. Sema3E. Sema3E regulates DC subsets. Higher numbers of CD11b + DC and lower numbers of CD103+ DC were detected in the lungs of Sema3E−/− mice at the steady-state condition and after allergen sensitization. The DC receptor involved in such Sema3E action is Plexin D1. c. Sema4A. Sema4A-mouse Tim2 (mTim2) or human ILT4 (hILT4) pathways costimulate T cells. Sema4A on DC directly binds mTim-2 or hILT4 on T cells. This leads to optimal T cell activation, proliferation and cytokine production. d. Sema4D. Distinct receptor-dependent effects of T cell-expressed Sema4D on DC functions. Sema4D costimulates T cells. Sema4D serves as an indirect costimulatory molecule for T cell activation. Sema4D on T cells stimulates DC to accelerate their activation and maturation. Stimulated DC, in their turn, enhance T cell activation. The main receptor for such Sema4D action is believed to be CD72. Sema4D costimulates DC. T cell-expressing and soluble Sema4D ligation of DC-expressing Plexin B1 and B2 receptors stimulates DC proinflammatory cytokine production and migration. e. Sema6D. Sema6D acts as indirect T cell costimulatory molecule. T cell expressed Sema6D activates DC through Plexin A1 receptor. Polyclonally- or Ag-stimulated T cells upregulate Sema6D expression. Sema6D stimulates T cell viability, proliferation and cytokine production on late stages of immune response. f. Sema7A. Sema7A in T cell-DC interaction. Indirect T cell stimulation by T cell expressed Sema7A ligation of Plexin C1 on DC.

In summary, these experiments indicated that sema3A is a potential novel therapeutic agent for the treatment of bronchial asthma.

Sema3E (originally termed M-SemaH) was first identified in the metastatic cell lines using a differential display technique which allowed to identify 2 splice variants encoding the same 775 a.a. protein [59]. The protein consists of a putative signaling sequence in NH- terminus followed by a large semaphorin domain, a c2 immunoglobulin-like domain at the amino acids 595–659, approximately 20 residues serving as a transmembrane domain, and positively charged residues in the COOH-terminus [59]. Sema3E contains 13 conserved cysteine residues and 3 potential A'-glycosylation sites. The amino acid sequence of Sema3E was found to be 82% identical to the reported partial sequence of chick collapsin 5 and 44–48% to all other members of the subclass III of the family [59]. Also, the AU-rich motif (AUUUA) conferring protein instability has been defined.

The extensive work by Movassagh and associates from the laboratory of Dr. Gounni at the University of Manitoba, Canada [60] defined the effect of Sema3E deficiency in experimental mouse model of asthma. Such deficiency resulted in substantial airway eosinophilia in untreated Sema3E$^{-/-}$ mice whereas the numbers of alveolar macrophages, T, B, NK, and NKT cells were comparable to those in WT mice. Therefore, the absence of Sema3E predisposed mice to allergic inflammation. Indeed, repeated inhalational exposure to HDM increased many components of asthmatic response in Sema3E$^{-/-}$ mice. This increase involved peribronchial inflammation, AHR to methacholine challenges, goblet cell hyperplasia, collagen deposition, and Th2/Th17 cytokine levels. All these features of asthmatic response were significantly downregulated when recombinant Sema3E was administered to the allergen sensitized mice intranasally [61]. A higher frequency of CD11b + pulmonary DC, a Th2- promoting subtype of DC, was observed in Sema3E−/− mice in both, the steady-state and allergen sensitized conditions as compared to WT control animals. When adoptively transferred to naïve mice, these Sema3E−/− CD11b + DC were able to induce the highest allergic lung inflammatory response especially when the DC recipients were Sema3E−/− mice. While examining the generated bone marrow chimeric mice, the authors defined the contribution of Sema3E on bone marrow-derived inflammatory cells in allergen-induced lung pathology. This work aligns with their previous study demonstrating Sema3E-mediated inhibition of human ASM cell proliferation and migration and defining the signaling pathways involved in such effect [62]. Moreover, their recent study clearly demonstrated a suppressed Sema3E expression in human severe asthma using bronchial biopsy and lung tissue histology specimens [63]. These data suggest that Sema3E plays an important regulatory role in allergic asthma. Targeting this molecule could be a novel approach to treat allergic asthma.

3.2 Sema4A and Sema4D

The Sema4A molecule is a 761 aa long glycoprotein of 150 kDa molecular weight with an NH2-terminal 32 aa signal peptide, a Sema domain, and an Ig domain of the C2 type (both 651 aa), a hydrophobic 21 aa transmembrane region, and a 57 aa cytoplasmic tail (Swissprot Accession # Q9H3S1). Its functions are the most complicated, diverse, and least studied. Sema4A has six known receptors (reviewed in 12). Sema4A exists in both membrane-bound and soluble forms [64, 65]. On the cell surface, it is expressed as a monomer and a dimer [65].

The role of Sema4A in asthma has been evaluated in the laboratory of Dr. Chapoval at the University of Maryland, USA [64, 66, 67]. It has been shown previously that lung-specific vascular endothelial growth factor (VEGF) expression induced asthma-like pathologies in the murine lungs [68, 69]. The experimental models of OVA-induced and VEGF-mediated allergic airway inflammation were used to assess the changes in expression of immune semaphorins and their receptors in mouse lung tissues [64]. We reported Sema4A expression was detected on bronchial epithelial cells, smooth muscle cells, and accessory-like cells. Both external allergen and lung local VEGF upregulated the expression of Sema4A and its receptors in the lung tissue. Allergen treatment led to a detection of a whole Sema4A protein plus its dimer in the bronchoalveolar (BAL) fluids under inflammation which was not found in the control mouse group. *In vivo* allergic response which consisted of eosinophilic BAL and lung tissue infiltration, mucous cell hyperplasia, AHR to methacholine challenges, sera Ag-specific IgG1/IgG2b/IgE contents, and IL-13 levels in BAL, sera, and cell cultures, was significantly upregulated in Sema4A−/− mice as compared to similarly treated WT mice [66]. In our next study, we employed *in vivo* re-introduction of rhSema4A to Sema4A-deficient and sufficient mice before the allergen challenge which was sufficient to downregulate the number of BAL eosinophils and the levels of BAL cytokines such as IL-6, IL-17A and TNFα [67]. Moreover, using rhSema4A in a chronic model of allergen exposure, we showed that it retains a potent anti-inflammatory effect even when lung tissue damage and remodeling are established [67]. The observed *in vivo* critical regulatory effect of Sema4A in acute and chronic allergic responses suggests that Sema4A-related pathways may be used for an immunotherapeutic asthma intervention.

A recent study by Lynch and associates [70] examined the role of Sema4A in respiratory syncytial virus (RSV)-induced bronchiolitis which is a predisposition for asthma. The authors used BDCA2-diphtheria toxin receptor (DTR) transgenic mice to induce the specific and reversible depletion of plasmacytoid DC (pDC) with intraperitoneal DT injections. They showed that pDC depletion in neonatal, but not adult, mice increased bronchiolitis severity and was sufficient to evoke an asthma-like phenotype upon viral challenge thus conforming that severe bronchiolitis in early life predisposes to subsequent asthma upon viral exposure. They also demonstrated that pDC from virus-infected mice expand Foxp3 + NRP1+ Treg cells and such expansion is effectively inhibited by the use of anti-Sema4A neutralizing Ab. Moreover, NRP1+ Treg cells transfer from infected to naïve mice prevents the recipients from viral bronchiolitis and subsequent asthma. This study further strengthens the importance of the Sema4A-mediated Treg cells expansion pathway and its important role in asthma protection and/or suppression.

Sema4D, also known as Cluster of Differentiation 100 (CD100), was the first semaphorin with defined expression and function in the immune system ([71, 72], reviewed in [12, 44, 73]). Several studies pointed to its critical regulatory role in the immune system ([74, 75], reviewed in [12, 44, 73, 76]). Sema4D consists of an NH2- terminal signal peptide, a sema domain, an Ig domain of the C2 type, a hydrophobic transmembrane region, and a cytoplasmic tail [71, 72]. The molecule's crystal modeling demonstrates the presence of a conserved seven-blade β-propeller structure [77] which is the structure of a conserved sema domain and is shared by all semaphorin family members. There is an 88% amino acid identity between human and murine Sema4D homologs [72]. Sema4D exists in both, membrane-bound and soluble forms, which are both biologically active [78, 79].

The recent report from Dr. Chapoval's laboratory at the University of Maryland has demonstrated an important regulatory role of Sema4D in asthma pathogenesis [80]. We exposed Sema4D-deficient and WT mice to OVA injections and challenges in the well-defined mouse model of OVA-induced experimental asthma. Sema4D-deficient mice demonstrated a significant decrease in eosinophilic airway infiltration after allergen challenge relative to WT mice. This reduced allergic inflammatory response was associated with decreased BAL Th2 and Th17 cytokine levels. The reduced T cell proliferation in $OVA_{323-339}$-restimulated Sema4D−/− cell cultures suggested lower T cell activation. Sema4D deficiency led to the increased number of Treg cells in mice after the allergen challenge. Surprisingly, Sema4D deficiency had no effect on airway hyperreactivity (AHR) to methacholine challenges in either acute or chronic experimental disease settings. Moreover, the lung DC number and activation were not affected by Sema4D deficiency. Our research data provided new insight into Sema4D biology and defined Sema4D as an important regulator of Th2-driven lung inflammation and as a potential target for disease immunotherapy.

3.3 Sema6D and Sema7A

Molecular cloning, mapping, and functional analysis of Sema6D together with Sema6C have been carried out more recently if compared to other semaphorins with costimulatory properties ([81], reviewed in [12]). Amino acid sequence alignment analysis of human semaphorin (HSA)SEMA6C, rat Sema6C, and mouse Sema6C showed the existence of the class VI semaphorin characteristic of the extracellular domain and PSI domain, which differ from all known members of semaphorin family. Predicted structure (HSA)SEMA6D isoforms were compared with related semaphorin proteins. Five isoforms of SEMA6D have been isolated and the significance of the alternatively spliced variants was evaluated by RT-PCR and Northern blots. The expression of different isoforms was found to be regulated in a tissue- and development-dependent manner. Sema6D consists of a signal peptide, a PSI domain, a transmembrane segment, an Ig domain, and a sema domain. Sequence analysis has shown that the translated polypeptides are composed of a 1–21 aa signal peptide followed by a 59–477 aa sema domain, a 508–563 aa PSI domain, a transmembrane segment, and a long cytoplasmic region.

The role of Sema6D in asthma has never been investigated. Based on the published data claiming a costimulatory role of Sema6D in T cell activation, we assume it regulates a disease severity. Regulation of T cell activation by Sema6D was examined *in vitro* and *in vivo* [82]. Upon T cell activation, after an initial decrease in Sema6D mRNA expression, they observed its stable upregulation and, later, a protein expression on the surface of T cells. This upregulation was relevant to both anti-CD3/CD28-stimulated and Ag-stimulated T cells. Using Sema6D-Ig, the authors identified Plexin A1 on DC as a Sema6D receptor. Interestingly, when anti-Sema6D blocking Ab was added to the cell cultures, it affected T cell proliferation in late stages (4–6 days of culture) whereas in the early stages (2–4 days), T cell viability and proliferation, as well as cytokine (IL-2) production, were not different from those without Ab in the culture. Specific targeting of Sema6D decreased T cell activation *in vivo* in the OTII cell adoptive transfer model. In this model, OTII T cells were obtained from the aTCR-transgenic strain that contains rearranged TCR-Vα and -Vβ genes in the germline DNA encoding a TCR specific for chicken ovalbumin (OVA) peptide 323–339 bound to I-A molecules in a context of H-2b haplotype (CD45.2). These CD45.2 cells were adoptively transferred to congenic B6-Ly5.2/Cr (CD45.1) recipients. The splenocyte proliferation was assessed as an expansion of donor OTII T cells in the recipient mice and expressed as the percentage of TCR+ CD4+ CD45.2+ cells in the isolated splenocyte population. The donor cell numbers were significantly lower when the recipient (CD45.1) mice received Sema6D-Ig at the time of cell plus OVA protein injections. Interestingly, Sema6D-Ig treatment did not affect an early T cell activation (day 4) but significantly reduced CD45.2+ T cell expansion on day 7. It is still unclear, however, if Plexin A1 is the only functional receptor for Sema6D on DC.

It is well established that macrophage polarization is a result of and a contributor to asthma pathogenesis [83]. Macrophages consist of more than 70% of lung cells and increased M2 macrophage polarization mirrored by increased Th2 response leads to further heightening of asthma pathology [83]. Macrophages and DCs expressed high levels of Sema6D [84]. Sema4D deficiency led to a downregulation of M2 polarization by bone marrow-derived macrophages accompanied by significant reductions in expression of Arg1, chitinase 3 like-1 (Chi3l1), Retnla, and Il10, as determined by qRT-PCR [84]. *In vivo*, Sema6D$^{-/-}$ mice demonstrated an exaggerated inflammatory response to LPS-induced sepsis accompanied by elevated levels of proinflammatory cytokines, including IL-12p40, TNF, and IL-6 as compared to WT mice. This study indirectly demonstrated the important role of Sema6D in asthma in part by regulation of macrophage polarization and activation.

The cDNA clone containing the entire coding sequence of the Sema7A gene and its molecular characteristics were first reported by Yamada and associates [85]. The human Sema7A cDNA clones were identified through the screening of a plasmid library generated from a leukemic T cell line. The 1998-base pairs of the cloned DNA's open reading frame encoded a 666 aa protein. This protein contained a 46 aa signal peptide and a 19 aa GPIanchor glycophosphatidylinositol linkage motif. The membrane-anchoring form of Sema7A was 602 aa long. The estimated molecular mass of the nonglycosylated form was 68 kDa. The authors located an "RGD (Arg-Gly-Asp) cell attachment sequence and the five potential N-linked glycosylation sites on the membrane-anchoring form". The expression of a native Sema7A form in transfected cells was confirmed by immunoprecipitation and flow cytometry analyses of cell transfectants. The Sema7A gene was identified on chromosome 15 (15q23–24) by radiation hybrid mapping. The 88.0% similarity at the nucleotide level was detected between murine and human Sema7A or 89.3% similarity at the amino acid level of corresponding proteins [86]. Both human and mouse SEMA7A contain a seven-bladed β-propeller semaphorin N- terminus domain, a plexin, semaphorin, and integrin domain (PSI), an immunoglobulin-like domain, and the characteristic for this particular semaphorin molecule GPI anchor in their C-terminus [87].

The extensive examination of a costimulatory function of Sema7A in T cell proliferation established this neuroimmune semaphorin as an inhibitor of T cell activation [88]. Sema7A$^{-/-}$ T cells demonstrated an enhanced proliferation upon Ag re-stimulation *in vitro*. However, no significant differences were observed in WT and Sema7A−/− DC maturation induced by various TLR ligands. Moreover, Sema7A deficiency in DC did not affect their ability to activate WT T cells. Furthermore, Sema7A$^{-/-}$ Treg cells were functional and actively comparably to WT Treg cells suppressed experimental colitis *in vivo*. This further points to a specific defect in the naive CD4 T cells associated with Sema7A deficiency. The proposed model of Sema7A function in T cell signaling is that Sema7A interacts with the components of the TCR complex and with a putative receptor on APCs which stabilizes TCR/CD3 complex and promotes inhibitory signals that limit T cell proliferation. The role of Sema7A in asthma has been reported in two recent publications [89, 90]. Sema7A was found to be expressed on the surface of circulating eosinophils and upregulated on bronchoalveolar lavage eosinophils obtained after segmental bronchoprovocation of asthmatic patients with allergen. Moreover, among all BAL cells, eosinophils were the predominant source of Sema7A. Among the members of the IL-5-family cytokines such as IL-3, IL-5, and GM-CSF, Sema7A protein on the surface of blood eosinophils was increased most by IL-3 exposure. The adherence of IL-3-activated eosinophils to the plate-bound receptor plexin C1 was doubled from the initial 30% in inactivated cells to 60% which proves the functional effect of Sema7A expressed on the eosinophil surface. Interestingly and relevant to asthma pathophysiology, a recombinant Sema7A induced alpha-smooth muscle actin production in human bronchial fibroblasts. These studies established semaphorin 7A as an important modulator of eosinophil profibrotic functions in the airway remodeling of patients

B7 family member	Role in asthma	Function	Reference
B7–1/B7–2	Stimulatory	Stimulates T cell activation and inflammatory cytokines production	[17, 18]
B7-H1 (PD-L1)/ B7-DC (PD-L2)	Inhibitory	Downregulates inflammatory cytokines production and airway hyperreactivity	[22, 25, 26]
B7-H2	Stimulatory	Induces Th2 cytokines and IgE productions	[28, 29]
B7-H3	Stimulatory	Increases Th2 and Th17 cytokine production	[35, 36]
B7-H4	Unknown		
B7-H5	Unknown		
B7-H6	Unknown		
B7-H7	Unknown		
ILDR2	Stimulatory	Promotes Th2 response	[42, 43]

Table 1.
Role of the B7 family members in asthma.

Semaphorin	Role in asthma	Function	Reference
Sema3A	Inhibitory	Stimulates Treg cells. Low serum levels correlate with asthma severity Downregulates lung inflammatory response	[55–58]
Sema3E	Inhibitory	Sema3E deficiency upregulates asthmatic response, led to a high frequency of Th2 promoting DC. Sema3E inhibits ASM cell proliferation. Low lung tissue expression is associated with higher asthma severity.	[60–63]
Sema4A	Inhibitory	Sema4A deficiency led to increases in many asthma parameters. Recombinant Sema4A applications *in vivo* led to a suppression of asthmatic response. Stimulates Treg cells *in vitro* and *in vivo*, induces new Treg cells in the *in vitro* CD4 + T cell cultures	[66, 67]
Sema4D	Stimulatory	Sema4D deficiency led to a lower lung inflammatory response to allergen challenges, lower T cell activation, and increased number of Treg cells	[80]
Sema6D	Unknown		
Sema7A	Inhibitory	Expressed on eosinophils. Regulates ASM contractility. Eosinophils are predominant source of Sema7A in the lungs. Lung Sema7A expression is upregulated by allergen bronchoprovocation	[89, 90]

Table 2.
Role of neuroimmune semaphorins in asthma.

with chronic asthma. The interference with the described pathway holds the potential to modulate asthma inflammation in the future (**Tables 1** and **2**).

4. Conclusions

Analysis of costimulatory molecules critically involved in asthma, a chronic respiratory Th2-driven disease, will help us to underline the immune mechanisms of disease development and progression. A complete understanding of these mechanisms will guide the development of novel therapeutic strategies to combat asthma and related allergies. Studies aimed to characterize the functions of several B7 family members and semaphorin family members in allergic asthma are either incomplete or ongoing. Further studies of the interplays between different individual costimulatory pathways should provide clearer insights into the disease pathology and guide the development of precise therapeutics.

Acknowledgements

S.P.C is supported by SemaPlex LLC and by NIH/NIAID RO1 AI076736 and RO1 AI143845 grants where she is a co-investigator. A.I.C. is supported by the Ministry of Science and Higher Education of the Russian Federation grant No. FZMW-2020-0007.

Author details

Svetlana P. Chapoval[1,2,3,4*] and Andrei I. Chapoval[5,6]

1 Department of Microbiology and Immunology, University of Maryland School of Medicine, Baltimore, MD, USA

2 Center for Vascular and Inflammatory Diseases, University of Maryland School of Medicine, Baltimore, MD, USA

3 Program in Oncology at the Greenebaum Cancer Center, University of Maryland School of Medicine, Baltimore, MD, USA

4 SemaPlex LLC, Ellicott City, MD, USA

5 Russian-American Anticancer Center, Altai State University, Barnaul, Russia

6 Center for Innovation in Medicine, Biodesign Institute, Arizona State University, Temple, AZ, USA

*Address all correspondence to: schapoval@som.umaryland.edu

References

[1] Chapoval SP, David CS. Identification of antigenic epitopes on human allergens: Studies with HLA transgenic mice. Environmental Health Perspectives. 2003;**111**(2):245-250

[2] Atamas SP, Chapoval SP, Keegan AD. Cytokines in chronic respiratory diseases. F1000 Biology Reports. 2013;**5**:3

[3] Tang ML, Khan MK, Croxford JL, Tan KW, Angeli V, Gasser S. The DNA damage response induces antigen presenting cell-like functions in fibroblasts. European Journal of Immunology. 2014;**44**(4):1108-1118

[4] Arebro J, Tengroth L, Razavi R, Kumlien Georén S, Winqvist O, Cardell LO. Antigen-presenting epithelial cells can play a pivotal role in airway allergy. The Journal of Allergy and Clinical Immunology. 2016;**137**(3): 957-60.e7

[5] Schuijs MJ, Hammad H, Lambrecht BN. Professional and 'Amateur' antigen-presenting cells In type 2 immunity. Trends in Immunology. 2019;**40**(1):22-34

[6] Esensten JH, Helou YA, Chopra G, Weiss A, Bluestone JA. CD28 Costimulation: From mechanism to therapy. Immunity. 2016;**44**(5):973-988

[7] Chapoval AI, Chapova SP, Shcherbakova NS, Shcherbakov DN. Immune checkpoints of the B7 family. Part 1. General characteristics and first representatives: B7-1, B7-2, B7-H1, B7-H2, and B7-DC. Russ. Journal of Bioorganic Chemistry. 2019;**45**:225-240

[8] Chapoval AI, Chapova SP, Shcherbakova NS, Shcherbakov DN. Immune checkpoints of the B7 family. Part 2. Representatives of the B7 family B7-H3, B7-H4, B7-H5, B7-H6, B7-H7, and ILDR2 and their receptors. Russ. Journal of Bioorganic Chemistry. 2019;**45**: 321-334

[9] Bhatia S, Edidin M, Almo SC, Nathenson SG. B7-1 and B7-2: Similar costimulatory ligands with different biochemical, oligomeric and signaling properties. Immunology Letters. 2006;**104**(1-2):70-75

[10] Kumanogoh A, Kikutani H. Roles of the semaphorin family in immune regulation. Advances in Immunology. 2003;**81**:173-198

[11] Yazdani U, Terman JR. The semaphorins. Genome Biology. 2006;**7**:211

[12] Chapoval SP. Neuroimmune semaphorins as costimulatory molecules and beyond. Molecular Medicine. 2018;**24**(1):13

[13] Yeganeh B, Xia C, Movassagh H, Koziol-White C, Chang Y, Al-Alwan L, et al. Emerging mediators of airway smooth muscle dysfunction in asthma. Pulmonary Pharmacology & Therapeutics. 2013;**26**(1):105-111

[14] Chapoval SP, Vadasz Z, Chapoval AI, Toubi E. Semaphorins 4A and 4D in chronic inflammatory diseases. Inflammation Research. 2017;**66**(2):111-117

[15] Kalmarzi RN, Rajabinejad M, Lotfi R. Immune semaphorins: Crucial regulatory signals and novel therapeutic targets in asthma and allergic diseases. European Journal of Pharmacology. 2020;**15**(881):173209

[16] Freeman GJ, Boussiotis VA, Anumanthan A, Bernstein GM, Ke XY, Rennert PD, et al. B7-1 and B7-2 do not deliver identical costimulatory signals, since B7-2 but not B7-1 preferentially costimulates the initial production of IL-4. Immunity. 1995;**2**:523-532

[17] Van Neerven RJ, Van de Pol MM, Van der Zee JS, Stiekema FE, De Boer M, Kapsenberg ML. Requirement of CD28-CD86 costimulation for allergen-specific T cell proliferation and cytokine expression. Clinical and Experimental Allergy. 1998;**28**:808-816

[18] Larche M, Till SJ, Haselden BM, North J, Barkans J, Corrigan CJ, et al. Costimulation through CD86 is involved in airway antigen-presenting cell and T cell responses to allergen in atopic asthmatics. Journal of Immunology. 1998;**161**:6375-6382

[19] Jaffar Z, Roberts K, Pandit A, Linsley P, Djukanovic R, Holgate S. B7 costimulation is required for IL-5 and IL-13 secretion by bronchial biopsy tissue of atopic asthmatic subjects in response to allergen stimulation. American Journal of Respiratory Cell and Molecular Biology. 1999;**20**:153-162

[20] Bellou A, Finn PW. Costimulation: Critical pathways in the immunologic regulation of asthma. Current Allergy and Asthma Reports. 2005;**5**:149-154

[21] Chen YQ, Shi HZ. CD28/CTLA-4--CD80/CD86 and ICOS--B7RP-1 costimulatory pathway in bronchial asthma. Allergy. 2006;**61**(1):15-26

[22] Bratke K, Fritz L, Nokodian F, Geißler K, Garbe K, Lommatzsch M, et al. Differential regulation of PD-1 and its ligands in allergic asthma. Clinical and Experimental Allergy. 2017;**47**(11): 1417-1425

[23] Akbari O, Stock P, Singh AK, et al. PD-L1 and PD-L2 modulate airway inflammation and iNKT-cell-dependent airway hyperreactivity in opposing directions. Mucosal Immunology. 2010;**3**:81-91

[24] Matsumoto K, Inoue H, Nakano T, et al. B7-DC regulates asthmatic response by an IFN-gamma-dependent mechanism. Journal of Immunology. 2004;**172**:2530-2541

[25] Oflazoglu E, Swart DA, Anders-Bartholo P, Jessup HK, Norment AM, Lawrence WA, et al. Paradoxical role of programmed death-1 ligand 2 in Th2 immune responses in vitro and in a mouse asthma model in vivo. European Journal of Immunology. 2004;**34**(12):3326-3336

[26] McAlees JW, Lajoie S, Dienger K, Sproles AA, Richgels PK, Yang Y, et al. Differential control of CD4(+) T-cell subsets by the PD-1/PD-L1 axis in a mouse model of allergic asthma. European Journal of Immunology. 2015;**45**(4):1019-1029

[27] Froidure A, Vandenplas O, D'Alpaos V, Evrard G, Pilette C. Persistence of asthma following allergen avoidance is associated with proTh2 myeloid dendritic cell activation. Thorax. 2015;**70**(10):967-973

[28] Hutloff A, Dittrich AM, Beier KC, Eljaschewitsch B, Kraft R, Anagnostopoulos I, et al. ICOS is an inducible T-cell co-stimulator structurally and functionally related to CD28. Nature. 1999;**397**:263-266

[29] Coyle AJ, Lehar S, Lloyd C, Tian J, Delaney T, Manning S, et al. The CD28-related molecule ICOS is required for effective T cell-dependent immune responses. Immunity. 2000;**13**(1): 95-105

[30] McAdam AJ, Chang TT, Lumelsky AE, Greenfield EA, Boussiotis VA, Duke-Cohan JS, et al. Mouse inducible costimulatory molecule (ICOS) expression is enhanced by CD28 costimulation and regulates differentiation of CD4+ T cells. Journal of Immunology. 2000;**165**(9):5035-5040

[31] Dong C, Juedes AE, Temann UA, Shresta S, Allison JP, Ruddle NH, et al. ICOS co-stimulatory receptor is essential for T-cell activation and function. Nature. 2001;**409**(6816): 97-101

[32] Uwadiae FI, Pyle CJ, Walker SA, Lloyd CM, Harker JA. Targeting the ICOS/ICOS-L pathway in a mouse model of established allergic asthma disrupts T follicular helper cell responses and ameliorates disease. Allergy. 2019;**74**(4):650-662

[33] Maazi H, Patel N, Sankaranarayanan I, Suzuki Y, Rigas D, Soroosh P, et al. ICOS:ICOS-ligand interaction is required for type 2 innate lymphoid cell function, homeostasis, and induction of airway hyperreactivity. Immunity. 2015;**42**(3):538-551

[34] Kadkhoda K, Wang S, Fan Y, Qiu H, Basu S, Halayko AJ, et al. ICOS ligand expression is essential for allergic airway hyperresponsiveness. International Immunology. 2011;**23**(4):239-249

[35] Chen ZR, Zhang GB, Wang YQ, Yan YD, Zhou WF, Zhu C, et al. Therapeutic effects of anti-B7-H3 antibody in an ovalbumin-induced mouse asthma model. Annals of Allergy, Asthma & Immunology. 2013;**111**(4):276-281

[36] Chen Z, Zhang G, Wang Y, Yan Y, Zhu C, Huang L, et al. B7-H3 expression in children with asthma exacerbation. Allergy and Asthma Proceedings. 2015;**36**(4):37-43

[37] Gu W, Zhang X, Yan Y, Wang Y, Huang L, Wang M, et al. B7-H3 participates in the development of asthma by augmentation of the inflammatory response independent of TLR2 pathway. Scientific Reports. 2017;**17**(7):40398

[38] Bhatt RS, Berjis A, Konge JC, Mahoney KM, Klee AN, Freeman SS, et al. KIR3DL3 is an inhibitory receptor for HHLA2 that mediates an alternative Immunoinhibitory pathway to PD1. Cancer Immunology Research. 2020;**9**(2):156-169

[39] Zhu Y, Yao S, Iliopoulou BP, Han X, Augustine MM, Xu H, et al. B7-H5 costimulates human T cells via CD28H. Nature Communications. 2013;**4**:2043

[40] Kaifu T, Escalière B, Gastinel LN, Vivier E, Baratin M. B7-H6/NKp30 interaction: A mechanism of alerting NK cells against tumors. Cellular and Molecular Life Sciences. 2011;**68**(21):3531-3539

[41] Dokmanovic-Chouinard M, Chung WK, Chevre JC, Watson E, Yonan J, Wiegand B, et al. Positional cloning of "Lisch-like", a candidate modifier of susceptibility to type 2 diabetes in mice. PLoS Genetics. 2008;**4**(7):e1000137

[42] Hecht I, Toporik A, Podojil JR, Vaknin I, Cojocaru G, Oren A, et al. ILDR2 is a novel B7-like protein that negatively regulates T cell responses. Journal of Immunology. 2018;**200**(6):2025-2037

[43] Gueguen C, Bouley J, Moussu H, Luce S, Duchateau M, Chamot-Rooke J, et al. Changes in markers associated with dendritic cells driving the differentiation of either TH2 cells or regulatory T cells correlate with clinical benefit during allergen immunotherapy. The Journal of Allergy and Clinical Immunology. 2016;**137**(2):545-558

[44] Nkyimbeng-Takwi E, Chapoval SP. Biology and function of neuroimmune semaphorins 4A and 4D. Immunologic Research. 2011;**50**(1):10-21

[45] Kolodkin AL, Matthes DJ, Goodman CS. The semaphorin genes encode a family of transmembrane and secreted growth cone guidance molecules. Cell. 1993;**75**:1389-1399

[46] Luo Y, Raible D, Raper JA. Collapsin: A protein in brain that induces the collapse and paralysis of neuronal growth cones. Cell. 1993;**75**:217-227

[47] Puschel AW, Adams RH, Betz H. Murine semaphorin D/collapsin is a

member of a diverse gene family and creates domains inhibitory for axonal extension. Neuron. 1995;**14**:941-948

[48] Polleux F, Morrow T, Ghosh A. Semaphorin 3A is a chemoattractant for cortical apical dendrites. Nature. 2000;**404**:567-573

[49] Antipenko A, Himanen JP, van Leyen K, Nardi-Dei V, Lesniak J, Barton WA, et al. Structure of the semaphorin-3A receptor binding module. Neuron. 2003;**39**(4):589-598

[50] Takahashi T, Fournier A, Nakamura F, Wang LH, Murakami Y, Kalb RG, et al. Plexin-neuropilin-1 complexes form functional semaphorin-3A receptors. Cell. 1999;**99**(1):59-69

[51] He Z, Tessier-Lavigne M. Neuropilin is a receptor for the axonal chemorepellent Semaphorin III. Cell. 1997;**90**:739-751

[52] Adams RH, Lohrum M, Klostermann A, Betz H, Puschel AW. The chemorepulsive activity of secreted semaphorins is regulated by furin-dependent proteolytic processing. The EMBO Journal. 1997;**16**:6077-6086

[53] Klostermann A, Lohrum M, Adams RH, Puschel AW. The chemorepulsive activity of the axonal guidance signal semaphorin D requires dimerization. The Journal of Biological Chemistry. 1998;**273**:7326-7331

[54] Lu D, Shang G, He X, Bai XC, Zhang X. Architecture of the Sema3A/PlexinA4/Neuropilin tripartite complex. Nature Communications. 2021;**12**(1):3172

[55] Cozacov R, Halasz K, Haj T, Vadasz Z. Semaphorin 3A: Is a key player in the pathogenesis of asthma. Clinical Immunology. 2017;**184**:70-72

[56] Toubi E, Vadasz Z. Semaphorin3A is a promising therapeutic tool for bronchial asthma. Allergy. 2020;**75**(2):481-483

[57] Adi SD, Eiza N, Bejar J, Shefer H, Toledano S, Kessler O, et al. Semaphorin 3A is effective in reducing both inflammation and angiogenesis in a mouse model of bronchial asthma. Frontiers in Immunology. 2019;**22**(10):550

[58] Sawaki H, Nakamura F, Aihara M, Nagashima Y, Komori-Yamaguchi J, Yamashita N, et al. Intranasal administration of semaphorin-3A alleviates sneezing and nasal rubbing in a murine model of allergic rhinitis. Journal of Pharmacological Sciences. 2011;**117**(1):34-44

[59] Christensen CR, Klingelhöfer J, Tarabykina S, Hulgaard EF, Kramerov D, Lukanidin E. Transcription of a novel mouse semaphorin gene, M-semaH, correlates with the metastatic ability of mouse tumor cell lines. Cancer Research. 1998;**58**:1238-1244

[60] Movassagh H, Shan L, Mohammed A, Halayko AJ, Gounni AS. Semaphorin 3E deficiency exacerbates airway inflammation, Hyperresponsiveness, and Remodeling in a mouse model of allergic asthma. Journal of Immunology. 2017;**198**:1805-1814

[61] Movassagh H, Shan L, Duke-Cohan JS, Halayko AJ, Uzonna JE, Gounni AS. Semaphorin 3E alleviates hallmarks of house dust mite-induced allergic airway disease. The American Journal of Pathology. 2017;**187**:1566-1576

[62] Movassagh H, Shan L, Halayko AJ, Roth M, Tamm M, Chakir J, et al. Neuronal chemorepellent Semaphorin 3E inhibits human airway smooth muscle cell proliferation and migration. The Journal of Allergy and Clinical Immunology. 2014;**133**(2):560-567

[63] Movassagh H, Shan L, Chakir J, McConville JF, Halayko AJ, Koussih L, et al. Expression of semaphorin 3E is suppressed in severe asthma. The Journal of Allergy and Clinical Immunology. 2017;**140**(4):1176-1179

[64] Smith EP, Shanks K, Lipsky MM, DeTolla LJ, Keegan AD, Chapoval SP. Expression of neuroimmune semaphorins 4A and 4D and their receptors in the lung is enhanced by allergen and vascular endothelial growth factor. BMC Immunology. 2011;**12**:30

[65] Toyofuku T, Yabuki M, Kamei J, Kamei M, Makino N, Kumanogoh A, et al. Semaphorin-4A, an activator for T-cell-mediated immunity, suppresses angiogenesis via Plexin-D1. The EMBO Journal. 2007;**26**(5):1373-1384

[66] Nkyimbeng-Takwi EH, Shanks K, Smith E, Iyer A, Lipsky MM, Detolla LJ, et al. Neuroimmune semaphorin 4A downregulates the severity of allergic response. Mucosal Immunology. 2012;**5**(4):409-419

[67] Mogie G, Shanks K, Nkyimbeng-Takwi EH, Smith E, Davila E, Lipsky MM, et al. Neuroimmune semaphorin 4A as a drug and drug target for asthma. International Immunopharmacology. 2013;**17**(3):568-575

[68] Lee CG, Link H, Baluk P, Homer RJ, Chapoval S, Bhandari V, et al. Vascular endothelial growth factor (VEGF) induces remodeling and enhances TH2-mediated sensitization and inflammation in the lung. Nature Medicine. 2004;**10**:1095-1103

[69] Bhandari V, Choo-Wing R, Chapoval SP, Lee CG, Tang C, Kim YK, et al. Essential role of nitric oxide in VEGF-induced, asthma-like angiogenic, inflammatory, mucus, and physiologic responses in the lung. Proceedings of the National Academy of Sciences of the United States of America. 2006;**103**(29): 11021-11026

[70] Lynch JP, Werder RB, Loh Z, Sikder MAA, Curren B, Zhang V, et al. Plasmacytoid dendritic cells protect from viral bronchiolitis and asthma through semaphorin 4a-mediated T reg expansion. The Journal of Experimental Medicine. 2018;**215**(2):537-557

[71] Hall KT, Boumsell L, Schultze JL, Boussiotis VA, Dorfman DM, Cardoso AA, et al. Human CD100, a novel leukocyte semaphorin that promotes B-cell aggregation and differentiation. Proceedings of the National Academy of Sciences of the United States of America. 1996;**93**(21): 11780-11785

[72] Furuyama T, Inagaki S, Kosugi A, Noda S, Saitoh S, Ogata M, et al. Identification of a novel transmembrane semaphorin expressed on lymphocytes. The Journal of Biological Chemistry. 1996;**271**(52):33376-33381

[73] Suzuki K, Kumanogoh A, Kikutani H. CD100/Sema4D, a lymphocyte semaphorin involved in the regulation of humoral and cellular immune responses. Cytokine & Growth Factor Reviews. 2003;**14**(1):17-24

[74] Bougeret C, Mansur IG, Dastot H, Schmid M, Mahouy G, Bensussan A, et al. Increased surface expression of a newly identified 150-kDa dimer early after human T lymphocyte activation. Journal of Immunology. 1992;**148**(2):318-323

[75] Herold C, Bismuth G, Bensussan A, Boumsell L. Activation signals are delivered through two distinct epitopes of CD100, a unique 150 kDa human lymphocyte surface structure previously defined by BB18 mAb. International Immunology. 1995;**7**:1-8

[76] Kumanogoh A, Kikutani H. Biological functions and signaling of a

transmembrane semaphorin, CD100/ Sema4D. Cellular and Molecular Life Sciences. 2004;**61**(3):292-300

[77] Love CA, Harlos K, Mavaddat N, Davis SJ, Stuart DI, Jones EY, et al. The ligand-binding face of the semaphorins revealed by the high-resolution crystal structure of SEMA4D. Nature Structural Biology. 2003;**10**:843-848

[78] Elhabazi A, Delaire S, Bensussan A, Boumsell L, Bismuth G. Biological activity of soluble CD100. I. the extracellular region of CD100 is released from the surface of T lymphocytes by regulated proteolysis. Journal of Immunology. 2001;**166**:4341-4347

[79] Zhu L, Bergmeier W, Wu J, Jiang H, Stalker TJ, Cieslak M, et al. Regulated surface expression and shedding support a dual role for semaphorin 4D in platelet responses to vascular injury. Proceedings of the National Academy of Sciences of the United States of America. 2007;**104**(5):1621-1626

[80] Shanks K, Nkyimbeng-Takwi EH, Smith E, Lipsky MM, DeTolla LJ, Scott DW, et al. Neuroimmune semaphorin 4D is necessary for optimal lung allergic inflammation. Molecular Immunology. 2013;**56**(4):480-487

[81] Qu X, Wei H, Zhai Y, Que H, Chen Q, Tang F, et al. Identification, characterization, and functional study of the two novel human members of the semaphorin gene family. The Journal of Biological Chemistry. 2002;**277**(38): 35574-35585

[82] O'Connor BP, Eun SY, Ye Z, Zozulya AL, Lich JD, Moore CB, et al. Semaphorin 6D regulates the late phase of CD4+ T cell primary immune responses. Proceedings of the National Academy of Sciences of the United States of America. 2008;**105**(35): 13015-13020

[83] Saradna A, Do DC, Kumar S, Fu QL, Gao P. Macrophage polarization and allergic asthma. Translational Research. 2018;**191**:1-14

[84] Kang S, Nakanishi Y, Kioi Y, Okuzaki D, Kimura T, Takamatsu H, et al. Semaphorin 6D reverse signaling controls macrophage lipid metabolism and anti-inflammatory polarization. Nature Immunology. 2018;**19**(6):561-570

[85] Yamada A, Kubo K, Takeshita T, Harashima N, Kawano K, Mine T, et al. Molecular cloning of a glycosylphosphatidylinositol-anchored molecule CDw108. Journal of Immunology. 1999;**162**(7):4094-4100

[86] Mine T, Harada K, Matsumoto T, Yamana H, Shirouzu K, Itoh K, et al. CDw108 expression during T-cell development. Tissue Antigens. 2000;**55**(5):429-436

[87] Liu H, Juo ZS, Shim AH, Focia PJ, Chen X, Garcia KC, et al. Structural basis of semaphorin-plexin recognition and viral mimicry from Sema7A and A39R complexes with PlexinC1. Cell. 2010;**142**(5):749-761

[88] Czopik AK, Bynoe MS, Palm N, Raine CS, Medzhitov R. Semaphorin 7A is a negative regulator of T cell responses. Immunity. 2006;**24**:591-600

[89] Esnault S, Kelly EA, Johansson MW, Liu LY, Han ST, Akhtar M, et al. Semaphorin 7A is expressed on airway eosinophils and upregulated by IL-5 family cytokines. Clinical Immunology. 2014;**150**(1):90-100

[90] Mizutani N, Nabe T, Yoshino S. Semaphorin 7A plays a critical role in IgE-mediated airway inflammation in mice. European Journal of Pharmacology. 2015;**764**:149-156

Chapter 2

Asthma and COVID-19

Gulfidan Uzan

Abstract

Asthma is a heterogeneous disease developed against various stimuli (indoor and outdoor allergens, cigarette, air pollution, etc.), associated with airway hypersensitivity and characterized by chronic airway inflammation. COVID-19 is a disease caused by a coronavirus strain called Severe Acute Respiratory Syndrome-coronavirus-2 (SARS-CoV-2). There may be some clinical confusions in proper diagnostics due to certain similarities of both diseases's symptoms such as, for example, a difficulty of breathing, cough, and shortness of breath. The current data on asthma being a risk factor for COVID-19 are controversial. It has been reported that asthma is not a risk factor for COVID-19 as the course of COVID-19 in patients with asthma is similar to that observed in the normal population. On the other hand, a current guidance from the World Health Organization (WHO) suggests that asthmatic patients can get more severe illness from COVID-19. Moreover, as with all respiratory tract infections, SARS-CoV-2 virus can certainly impair asthma control. However, recent studies suggest a potential beneficial effect of corticosteroids on SARS-CoV-2 infection as they suppress type II inflammation and restore anti-viral immunity. Prolonged use of a high dose of systemic steroids can increase susceptibility to infection and the occurrence of systemic side effects. However, patients with asthma should definitely continue their prescribed treatment with inhaler steroids and other additional medicines they use during SARS-CoV-2 infection. In asthmatic patients infected with SARS-CoV-2, the most significant risk factor is the loss of asthma control and subsequent presentation to healthcare centers due to the lack of asthma control. Therefore, the asthmatic patients using biological agents are recommended to continue their prescribed treatment such as omelizumab, mopelizumab and prolong the treatment intervals during the peak of infection.

Keywords: asthma, COVID-19, pandemic, asthma treatment, inflammation

1. Introduction

COVID-19 is a disease caused by a novel *coronavirus strain* [1–10], which has been named by the *International Committee on Taxonomy of Viruses* (ICTV) as SARS-CoV-2. It has caused a severe viral pandemic worldwide since March 2020 [8, 11]. The virus was first reported in Wuhan, China. Its source is thought to be a live animal market, namely bats [12]. The transmission is via respiratory droplets [8, 9]. The mean incubation period is 2 to 7 days and the main symptoms include fatigue, shortness of breath, fever, coughing, loss of smell and taste, sore throat, muscle pain, headache, vomiting and diarrhea [2, 13]. The course of disease is highly variable. Comorbidities seen in infected individuals are important in terms of the healing time, going to intensive care, and affecting mortality. Among these comorbidities, particular conditions such as hypertension, ischemic heart diseases, diabetes, and chronic obstructive pulmonary disease represent the most important risk factors for a severe course of disease [13, 14].

Asthma is one of the most common chronic respiratory tract diseases [15]. It is considered to affect approximately 300 million people across the world. Prevalence rates vary to a great extent, ranging from 1% to 18% in children and adults in different countries [16]. Asthma exacerbation is an important reason for emergency admission [15, 16]. It is defined by respiratory symptoms such as wheezing, shortness of breath, tightness in the chest and/or coughing and expiratory air flow limitation. These signs vary in in time. Usually, exacerbations are observed due to various factors like allergy or irritants, exercise, change of air or respiratory tract infections. Symptoms and airway limitation are frequently resolved with treatment or spontaneously and may be absent for weeks or months. On the other hand, such exacerbations may be life-threatening, i.e. the disease may have various clinical presentations and severities which are specific to each patient [16]. For an effective treatment and control of the disease, it is important to educate the patient and help to cooperate with the doctor. The education includes preparation of a written asthma action plan and medical evaluation at regular intervals. A written asthma action plan is a document prepared specifically for the patient by the doctor to show how to monitor his/her symptoms and respiratory functions at home, and it should be reviewed by the physician at regular intervals. This plan helps the patients recognize the aggravation of their asthma and use suitable treatment options [16]. This is very important for minimizing asthmatic patients' visits to healthcare centers during the pandemic and decreasing the risk of transmission [16, 17].

In pandemic the patients with asthma should be managed in two groups: the patients who have asthma but have not yet contracted COVID-19, and those who have asthma and have contracted COVID-19 [18]. COVID-19 and subsequent association between asthma and COVID-19 is a challenging clinical condition with more questions than answers. However, we can make some predictions based on the available data.

2. Management of a patient with asthma who has not contracted COVID-19

The main objective for patients should be to avoid COVID-19 infection. At first, the patient should be informed that asthma does not pose an extra risk for contracting COVID-19 as well as leading to a severe course of disease [19, 20]. Social isolation and adherence to hygiene rules are the most important factors in prevention of disease transmission. Patients with asthma are recommended to remain isolated in their home environment, if possible. They should be instructed to self-monitor symptoms using a PEFmeter [21]. Thus, visits to healthcare centers should be kept at minimum. If patients do not have serious problems during this period, scheduled visits should be delayed as much as possible and physicians should be consulted by telephone, if necessary. In case of any increase in coughing and/or shortness of breath, first of all, it should be made sure that the bronchodilators are delivered at adequate doses and the bronchodilator device (nebulizer) is used correctly. The patients should be instructed by their physician about what to do when their asthma gets worse by means of a written action plan. Considering that an asthma patient who1 is on a control-visit may be a potential COVID-19 carrier, it is very important not to perform a respiratory function test unless it is extremely necessary. Otherwise, it is recommended to keep the room very well ventilated, provide the test technician with appropriate protective equipment, particularly an N95 mask, and perform the test in a negative pressure room, if possible [22].

Approximately 80% of patients with asthma have allergic rhinitis and approximately 40% of patients with allergic rhinitis have allergic asthma. It is important to keep the symptoms of allergic rhinitis under control for control of asthma [22–24]. Patients with allergic rhinitis can also use their nasal steroids and antihistamines safely during this pandemic [23, 25]. During the quarantine, patients may have trouble gaining access to their medications due to outgoing restrictions and risk of contamination. In Turkey, the validity of the medication reports for patients with asthma has been extended from March 1st, 2020 by the Turkish Ministry of Health and Social Security Institution so that patients can obtain their medicines from pharmacies without prescription [8]. The validity of disability reports has been also automatically extended. If patients with allergic rhinitis do not use their drugs for symptom control especially during the pollen season, their sneezing will increase. The same also applies for patients allergic to house dust mites. Spring time poses a risk for asthma attacks in patients with pollen allergy while similarly prolonged isolation and quarantine is a risk factor for an attack and loss of asthma control in asthma patients allergic to house dust mites. If patients with pollen allergy follow the rules of isolation and avoid going out, their symptoms will be under control due to reduced contact with pollens. These patients should ventilate their rooms in the afternoon and, if they have to ventilate it in the morning, they should stay in another room. In patients with allergic rhinitis who use masks effectively when they go out, exposure to pollens will be reduced and thus their symptoms and the need for medications will also be decreased. Patients with allergic rhinitis sensitized to house dust mites are unfortunate during this period because of a prolonged stay in closed environments. Therefore, it is very important that they use their allergic rhinitis medications regularly and follow the measures to protect themselves from house dust mites. While hand disinfectants containing chlorhexidine are not effective in SARS-CoV-2 [26], they may also lead to asthma attacks in those allergic to this chemical [26]. Use of latex hand gloves for hand hygiene may also lead to asthma attacks in patients with latex allergy, therefore the washing hands with soap and water should be preferred [26].

As a result asthma patients who have not contracted COVID-19 should definitely continue their inhaler steroid treatments and additional prescribed medications, and should follow the protection and hygiene rules as much as possible even when they are clinically stable [8, 16]. Discontinuation of controlling medications leads to disease exacerbation, increases the risk of having an asthma attack and eventually poses a higher risk for SARS CoV-2 contamination by hospital admission. Doses of inhaler steroids should not be reduced even when asthma is under control. The disease may also be controlled with non-steroidal treatments in some patients with asthma. In these patients, other treatments should be continued without steroids or in combination with low dose steroids [18]. Systemic steroids should be used as short as possible in patients with severe asthma. Because in long-term use, susceptibility to infection and steroid side effects may occur [15, 18].

3. Management of a patient with asthma who has contracted COVID-19

Pathophysiology of the coronaviruses (CoVs) and asthma comorbidity is complex and many aspects are unknown. In this book chapter we review the available literature on the pathogenesis of asthma and COVID-19.

Asthma is characterized by chronic airway inflammation [16], mainly a type 2 inflammation. Type 2 immunity involves helper T cells (Th 2), type 2 B cells, type 2 innate lymphoid cells, type 2 macrophages, IL-4 releasing natural killer (NK) and natural killer T (NKT) cells, basophils, eosinophils and mast cells [3, 4]. In general, antiviral and allergic responses are two separate branches of immunity and interact in a comprehensive network of interactions. Type I IFNs are the family of antiviral cytokines that play an important and central role in this network. In asthma, release of type I IFNs from bronchial epithelial cells and plasmacytoid dendritic cells is disrupted [3, 4].

It is well known that eosinophils play a central role in allergic diseases including asthma [4]. The possible effects of eosinophils on CoV are also remarkable. Eosinophils have a potential role in enhancing viral clearance and antiviral host defense. Recombinant eosinophil-derived neurotoxin (a major eosinophil ribonuclease) is capable of reducing the infectivity of respiratory syncytial virus (RSV). In addition, eosinophils can be activated with ssRNA through triggering the TLR-7-MyD88 signaling pathway, which might result in RSV clearance and limitation of virus-induced lung dysfunction. The low prevalence of COVID-19 in asthma patients may be due to eosinophils' defense against the virus. Eosinopenia occurs in COVID-19, pathophysiology is unclear [27]. Blockade of eosinophil release from bone marrow during acute infection, decreased expression of chemokine receptors or direct eosinophil apoptosis may caused by type 1 IFNs may be responsible. There is little indication that eosinophils play a protective or aggravating role during SARS-CoV-2 infection. Eosinopenia, however, may be a prognostic indicator for more severe SARS-CoV-2 infection [27]. Additionally, it is not known whether eosinopenia is a consequence of impaired immunity or biologics intake. The role of eosinophils in the course of eosinophilic inflammation associated with SARS-CoV-2 infection and allergy needs to be investigated further [4].

In theory, asthma as a lung-targeted chronic disease should increase the vulnerability of lung tissue to COVID-19 infection and should lead to a worse course of COVID-19 and reduced anti-viral immune response. But, interestingly, it was reported that asthma produces a type 2 inflammatory cytokines (IL-4,-5 and − 13) and accumulation of eosinophils in the airways and their number increases systemically, what provides a protection against COVID-19 [4]. As with SARS and other seasonal coronaviruses, SARS-Cov-2 also uses the cellular receptors of angiotensin converting enzyme 2 (ACE2) to invade the cells. Upregulated ACE-2 expression increases the sensitivity of receptor-expressing cells to infection. However, ACE-2 expression in the respiratory tract epithelium is decreased in patients with asthma as compared to normal control subjects, and this protects from COVID-19 [4, 5, 28]. Allergic diseases do not predispose to COVID-19 and does not increase COVID-19 severity. Asthma also does not pose a risk to COVID-19, and there is no difference between asthma patients with and without COVID-19 in terms of hospital admission and severity of the course of disease [15, 28–30]. When patients with asthma contract COVID-19, they have a disease course similar to that of the normal population [15, 31]. But as with all viruses causing respiratory tract infections, SARS-CoV-2 is also a risk factor for asthma attacks and disrupts asthma control [16, 32]. Despite proper and adequate treatment bronchodilator therapy, patients with increased symptoms, additional symptoms and/or contact history should be admitted to the hospital and undergo appropriate examination and investigations.

Exacerbation of asthma and allergic rhinitis may also be confused with COVID-19 clinically [8, 23]. Dry coughs and shortness of breath may be seen asthma, allergic rhinitis and COVID-19. Seasonality of symptoms and history of symptom development in the presence of exposure to a certain allergic agent are quite helpful in the differential diagnosis of allergic rhinitis. Atopy test also supports the diagnosis. It is also very important to distinguish between an asthma attack and COVID-19 infection attack in a patient with a prior diagnosis of asthma as both display interfering symptoms such as shortness of breath and coughing. Therefore, differential diagnosis is extremely significant in the group of patients with such comorbidity.

In addition to the clinical presentation, laboratory findings (such as eosinophil and lymphocyte count, C reactive protein, D Dimer) may also be beneficial in the differential diagnosis. While presence of lymphopenia and eosinopenia in hemogram may favor COVID-19 [8] increased eosinophil levels may indicate asthma. While an asthma patient presenting with symptoms such as coughing, shortness of breath, wheezing and stridor without any additional finding should be primarily evaluated for an asthma attack; considering that everybody may be infected in such a pandemic, extra care should be exercised regarding social isolation, distance and the use of personal protective equipment for the safety of both patient and healthcare personnel [8]. Asthmatic patients who develop weakness, loss of smell and taste should have chest X-ray and blood tests for COVID-19 [8].

4. Symptoms of asthma, COVID-19 and allergic rhinitis

Corticosteroids hold a significant place in the treatment of asthma [2]. High-dose corticosteroids have been used α during the SARS and MERS outbreaks and in COVID-19 to suppress lung inflammation during critical illness of infected patients. Corticosteroids (inhaled or systemic) can inhibit production of the critical antiviral mediators type I and III interferons [3]). At the same time its suppress type 2 inflammation and their use in COVID-19-associated exacerbation may lead to the beneficial effect of secondary restoration of impaired antiviral immunity. However, clinical evidence of corticosteroid use in COVID-19 is still insufficient [3].

In patients with asthma who have contracted COVID-19, inhaled corticosteroid dose may be increased 4-fold depending on the severity of the disease or use of systemic administration of steroids is recommended [18, 30]. In patients with severe asthma, systemic steroid therapy should be used as short as possible, as in asthma patients without COVID-19.

Steroid therapy preferably should be taken in the form of metered-dose inhalers containing dry powder rather than nebulizers [5, 33]. Metered-dose inhalers are ideal devices thanks to their ease of use and low risk of viral transmission, but they may not be effective in cases of severe dyspnea, cognitive or neuromuscular disorders and respiratory failure with inadequate inspiratory strength [33]. Dry powder inhalers are able to reach the lungs in low inspiratory flow and do not require hand-breath coordination (squeezing the inhaler medication at the same time while breathing deeply). On the other hand, dry powder inhalers may lead to irritation in the airways and coughing, and a by creating aerolization potential viral transmission is also of question. It is contradictory whether the treatment with a nebulizer is risky in terms of viral transmission due to aerosolization [34]. As a result, a metered-dose inhalator with a valved reservoir or dry powder inhaler is preferred for reducing the auto-aerosolization and spread of the virus [35].

Leukotriene receptor antagonists with their beneficial anti-inflammatory and bronchodilator activities may also be added to the treatment of the patients with COVID-19 and asthma admitted to the hospital [5, 30, 36].

Azithromycin has been shown to be an effective treatment in decreasing the frequency of exacerbations and improving the quality of life in asthma patients whose condition cannot be controlled with standard treatment [31, 37]. Azithromycin decreases the risk of COVID-19-related severe outcomes by increasing the IFN production associated with a natural antiviral immunity in respiratory tract cells [37]. However, azithromycin is not recommended for prophylactic treatment of COVID-19 [37].

An asthma patient receiving allergen immunotherapy who is infected with COVID-19 or in contact with an infected person may continue to receive his/her treatment in the absence of any symptoms [38]. It has been reported that immune response to virus can be improved and cytokine storm can be prevented by this treatment [4, 30, 39]. But if there are any signs of respiratory tract infection, it is recommended to treat this infection [39].

Use of Anti-IgE, anti-IL-5/IL-5 alfa, anti-IL-4 alfa is not risky for patient with asthma who has contracted COVID-19, therefore such medications may be safely used to control asthma [30, 40]. Although patients using biologic agents are recommended to continue their treatment. During the period of COVID-19 peak, biological agent treatment is applied less frequently. Biological agent therapy continues as before when symptoms are improved or COVID-PCR becomes negative [22, 23]. Since patients with severe asthma may be at higher risk of severe COVID-19 infection, they should avoid any activities which may disrupt their asthma control and they should use their asthma therapies properly.

In conclusion, asthma does not represent a risk factor for COVID-19 and asthma does not adversely affect the course of COVID-19. However, it is extremely important to keep asthma under control particularly during the pandemic period. Patients with asthma should be recommended to continue to use inhaler steroids that keep their asthma under control along with other prescribed medications. Patients should be provided with a written emergency action plan because nowadays a visit to a healthcare center carries a risk for the SARS-CoV-2 infection. In order to prevent the risk of transmission of infection, training should be given on maintaining social isolation and distance, avoiding contact, hand hygiene and correct use of masks.

Author details

Gulfidan Uzan
Department of Chest Disease, University of Health Science, Sultangazi Haseki Training and Research Hospital, Istanbul, Turkey

*Address all correspondence to: gulfidan70@gmail.com

References

[1] Kumar K, Hinks TSC, Singanayagam A. Treatment of COVID-19-exacerbated asthma: should systemic corticosteroids be used? Am J Physiol Lung Cell Mol Physiol. 2020 Jun 1;318(6):L1244-L1247. doi: 10.1152/ajplung.00144.2020. Epub 2020 May 13. PMID: 32401670; PMCID: PMC7276980.

[2] Chhiba KD, Patel GB, Vu THT, Chen MM, Guo A, Kudlaty E, Mai Q, Yeh C, Muhammad LN, Harris KE, Bochner BS, Grammer LC, Greenberger PA, Kalhan R, Kuang FL, Saltoun CA, Schleimer RP, Stevens WW, Peters AT. Prevalence and characterization of asthma in hospitalized and nonhospitalized patients with COVID-19. J Allergy Clin Immunol. 2020 Aug;146(2):307-314. e4. doi: 10.1016/j.jaci.2020.06.010. Epub 2020 Jun 15. PMID: 32554082; PMCID: PMC7295471.

[3] Liu S, Cao Y, Du T, Zhi Y. Prevalence of Comorbid Asthma and Related Outcomes in COVID-19: A Systematic Review and Meta-Analysis. J Allergy Clin Immunol Pract. 2020 Dec 9:S2213-2198(20)31328-3. doi: 10.1016/j.jaip.2020.11.054. Epub ahead of print. PMID: 33309934; PMCID: PMC7725230.

[4] Liu S, Zhi Y, Ying S. COVID-19 and asthma: reflection during the pandemic. Clin Rev Allergy Immunol. 2020; 59:78-88.

[5] Alexzandra Hughes-Visentin, and Anthea B Mahesan Paul. Asthma and COVID-19: What do we know now? Clinical Medicine Insights: Circulatory, Respiratory and Pulmonary Medicine. 2020;14: 1-7.

[6] World Health Organization. Director-General's remarks at the media briefing on 2019-nCoV on 11 February 2020. https://www.who.int/dg/speeches/detail/who director generals remarks at the media briefing on 2019 ncov on 11-february-2020.

[7] Stanbury RM, Graham EM. Systemic corticosteroid therapy—side effects and their management Br J Ophthalmol 1998;82:704-708. http://dx.doi.org/10.1136/bjo.82.6.704

[8] Turkish Respiratory Society. Coronavirüs hastalığı, 2019(COVID-19) ve akciğer: Göğüs hastalıkları uzmanlarının bilmesi gerekenler. Ozseker ZF. Chapter 2: Astım ve COVID-19. Eurasian Journal of Pulmonology. 2020:92-96. in Turkish.

[9] Coronaviridae Study Group of the International Committee on Taxonomy of Viruses. The species severe acute respiratory syndrome-related coronavirus: classifying 2019-nCoV and naming it SARSCoV-2. Nat Microbiol 2020; 5:536-544.

[10] Lu R, Zhao X, Li J, Niu P, Yang B, Wu H, et al. Genomic characterisation and epidemiology of 2019 novel coronavirus: implications for virus origins and receptor binding. Lancet 2020;395: 565-574.

[11] Li X, Xu S, Yu M, Wang K, Tao Y, Zhou Y, et al. Risk factors for severity and mortality in adult COVID-19 inpatients in Wuhan. J Allergy Clin Immunol. July 2020;146(1):110-118.

[12] Chen N, Zhou M, Dong X, Qu J, Gong F, Han Y, et al. Epidemiological and clinical char-acteristics of 99 cases of 2019 novel coronavirus pneumonia in Wuhan, China: a de-scriptive study. Lancet 2020; 395:507-513.

[13] Guan WJ, Ni ZY, Hu Y, Liang WH, Ou CQ, He JX, et al. Clinical characteristics of coronavirus disease 2019 in China. N Engl J Med 2020; 382:1708-1720

[14] ECDC. Outbreak of novel coronavirus disease 2019 (COVID-19): increased transmission globally-fifth update. https://www.ecdc.europa.eu/sites/default/files/documents/RRA-outbreak-novel-coronavirusdisease-2019-increase-transmission-globally-COVID- 19.pdf. 96

[15] Chhiba KD, Patel GB, Vu THT, Chen MM, Guo A, Kudlaty E, et al. Prevalence and characterization of asthma in hospitalized and nonhospitalized patients with COVID-19. J Allergy Clin Immunol. 2020 Aug;146(2):307-314.e4. doi: 10.1016/j.jaci.2020.06.010. Epub 2020 Jun 15. PMID: 32554082; PMCID: PMC7295471.

[16] Turkish Thoracic Journal. Official Journal of Turkish Thoracic Society. Asthma Guideline. Supplement 01October 2016. Volume 17.

[17] Oreskovic NM, Kinane BT, Aryee E, Kuhlthau KA, Perrin JM. The Unexpected Risks of COVID-19 on Asthma Control in Children, J Allergy Clin Immunol Pract. 2020;8(8):2489-2491. ISSN 2213-2198, https://doi.org/10.1016/j.jaip.2020.05.027

[18] Syed Shahzad Hasan, Toby Capstick, Syed Tabish Razi Zaidi, Chia Siang Kow, Hamid A. Merchant. Use of corticosteroids in asthma and COPD patients with or without COVID-19. Respiratory Medicine 170 (2020) 106045.

[19] Zhang JJ, Dong X, Cao YY, Yuan YD, Yang YB, Yan YQ, et al. Clinical characteristics of 140 patients infected with SARS-CoV-2 in Wuhan, China. Allergy 2020;10.1111/all.14238.

[20] Dong X, Cao YY, Lu XX, Zhang JJ, Du H, Yan YQ, et al. Eleven faces of coronavirus disease 2019. Allergy 2020;10.1111/all.14289.

[21] Asthma GIf. COVID-19: GINA ANSWERS TO FREQUENTLY ASKED QUESTIONS ON ASTHMA MANAGEMENT. 2020; https://ginasthma.org/covid-19-gina-answers-to-frequentlyasked-questions-on-asthma-management/. Accessed May 21, 2020.

[22] Global Initiatives for Asthma. Global Strategy for Asthma Management and Prevention 2020, www.ginasthma.org

[23] Shaker MS, Oppenheimer J, Grayson M, Stukus D, Hartog N, Hsieh EWY, et al. COVID-19: Pandemic contingency planning for the allergy and immunology clinic. J Allergy Clin Immunol Pract 2020; S2213-2198(20)30253-1. doi: 10.1016/j.jaip.2020.03.012.

[24] Bousquet J, Khaltaev N, Cruz AA, Denburg J, Fokkens WJ, Togias A, et al. Allergic rhinitis and its impact on asthma (ARIA) 2008 update (in collaboration with World Health Or-ganization, GALLEN and AllerGen). Allergy 2008; 63:8-160.

[25] Bousquet J, Akdis C, Jutel M, Bachert C, Klimek L, Agache I, et al. ARIA-MASK study group. Intranasal corticosteroids in allergic rhinitis in COVID-19 infected patients: An ARIA-EAACI statement. Allergy 2020;10.1111/all.14302.

[26] Kelly KJ, Sussman G. Latex allergy: Where are we now and how did we get there? J Allergy Clin Immunol Pract 2017; 5:1212-1216.

[27] Lindsley AW, Schwartz JT, Rothenberg ME, Eosinophil responses during COVID-19 infections and coronavirus vaccination, J Allergy Clin Immunol. 2020;146(1): 1-7. ISSN 0091-6749, https://doi.org/10.1016/j.jaci.2020.04.021.

[28] Jackson DJ, Busse WW, Bacharier LB, et al. Association of respiratory allergy, asthma, and

expression of the SARS-CoV-2 receptor ACE2. J Allergy Clin Immunol. 2020; 146:203-206.

[29] Zhu Z, Hasegawa K, Ma B, Fujiogi M, Camargo CA, Liang L. Association of asthma and its genetic predisposition with the risk of severe COVID-19. J Allergy Clin Immunol. 2020; 146:327-329.

[30] Liu S, Cao Y, Du T, Zhi Y. Prevalence of Comorbid Asthma and Related Outcomes in COVID-19: A Systematic Review and Meta-Analysis. J Allergy Clin Immunol Pract. 2020 Dec 9:S2213-2198(20)31328-3. doi: 10.1016/j.jaip.2020.11.054. Epub ahead of print. PMID: 33309934; PMCID: PMC7725230

[31] Riggioni C, Comberiati P, Giovannini M, Agache I, Akdis A. A compendium answering 150 questions on COVID-19 and SARS-CoV-2. Allerg. 2020 Oct;75(10):2503-2541. doi: 10.1111/all.14449. Epub 2020 Jul 20.

[32] Abrams E, Jong G, Yang C. Paediatric asthma and COVID-19. Ottawa: Canadian Paediatric Society; 2020 Apr. 1. Available:www.cps.ca/en/documents/position/paediatric-asthma -and-covid-19 (Erişim Tarihi: 21 Nisan 2020).

[33] Ari A. Promoting safe and effective use of aerosol devices in COVID-19: risks and suggestions for viral transmission. Expert Opin Drug Deliv. 2020. doi:10.1080/17425247.2020.1811225.

[34] Wan G-H, Tsai Y-H, Wu Y-K, Tsao K-C. A large-volume nebulizer would not be an infectious source for severe acute respiratory syndrome. Infect Control Hosp Epidemiol. 2004; 25:1113-1115.

[35] Licskai C, Yang CL, Ducharme FM, et al. Addressing therapeutic questions to help Canadian physicians optimize asthma management for their patients during the COVID-19 pandemic. Can J Respir Crit Care Sleep Med. 2020; 4:73-76.

[36] Khan A, Misdary C, Yegya-Raman N, et al. Montelukast in hospitalized patients diagnosed with COVID-19. 2020. doi:10.21203/rs.3.rs-52430/v1.30. Johnston SL. Asthma and COVID-19: is asthma a risk factor for severe outcomes? Allergy. 2020; 75:1543-1545.

[37] Lane JC, Weaver J, Kostka K, et al. Safety of hydroxychloroquine, alone and in combination with azithromycin, in light of rapid wide-spread use for COVID-19: a multinational network cohort and self-controlled case series study. medRxiv. 2020.

[38] Sajuthi SP, DeFord P, Jackson ND, et al. Type 2 and interferon inflammation strongly regulate SARS-CoV-2 related gene expression in the airway epithelium. Biorxiv. 2020

[39] Klimek L, Jutel M, Akdis C, et al. Handling of allergen immunotherapy in the COVID-19 pandemic: an ARIA-EAACI statement. Allergy. 2020;75:1546-1554.

[40] Mário Morais-Almeida, Rita Aguiara, Bryan Martin, Ignacio J. Ansoteguic, Motohiro Ebisawad, L. Karla Arrudae, et al. COVID-19, asthma, and biological therapies: What we need to know. World Allergy Organization Journal (2020) 13:100126 http://doi.org/10.1016/j.waojou.2020.100126

Chapter 3

Personalized Digital Phenotype Score, Healthcare Management and Intervention Strategies Using Knowledge Enabled Digital Health Framework for Pediatric Asthma

Utkarshani Jaimini and Amit Sheth

Abstract

Asthma is a personalized, and multi-trigger respiratory condition which requires continuous monitoring and management of symptoms and medication adherence. We developed kHealth: Knowledge-enabled Digital Healthcare Framework to monitor and manage the asthma symptoms, medication adherence, lung function, daily activity, sleep quality, indoor, and outdoor environmental triggers of pediatric asthma patients. The kHealth framework collects up to 1852 data points per patient per day. It is practically impossible for the clinicians, parents, and the patient to analyze this vast amount of multimodal data collected from the kHealth framework. In this chapter, we describe the personalized scores, clinically relevant asthma categorization using digital phenotype score, actionable insights, and potential intervention strategies for better pediatric asthma management.

Keywords: Pediatric patients, Asthma management, Multimodal data, Personalization, Intervention, Digital phenotype, Actionable information, Self monitoring, Self management

1. Introduction

Asthma is a multi-trigger disease with or without co-morbities such as obstructive sleep apnea, increase in body mass index (BMI), rhinitis, sinusitis, gastroesophageal reflux disease, psychopathologies etc. [1]. 8.3% of children in United States suffer from asthma [2]. Pediatric asthma affects the child's quality of life with reduced activity, lack of concentration, growing up with missed school days, emergency room visits, etc. [3].

As per the current clinical practice, the clinician does not get the holistic view of the asthma patient's health condition during the clinic visit scheduled once in every one to two months for severe persistent and once in six months for mild persistent asthma patient [4]. However, with the advent of Internet of Things (IoTs) sensors and mobile applications for collecting Patient Generated Health Data (PGHD) it has become convenient for patients (parents in the case of children below age 12) to log their daily symptoms, medication intake, and daily activity. The multi-modal

IntechOpen

PGHD is big data which suffers from challenges of velocity, volume, and variety [5]. The data is collected at different intervals for each sensor, is of different variety and volume. It is challenging to integrate this overwhelming data for analysis. It is impossible for the clinicians alone to analyze this data coming in with different velocity, variety, and volume along with their existing duties. It is challenging and practically impossible for the clinicians and the patients to generate actionable insights from this vast amount of data due to lack of time, resources, and data analysis skills [6].

In this chapter, we introduce a knowledge enabled healthcare framework, kHealth, which is being used by the pediatric asthma patients for self monitoring and by the clinicians to derive real time insights into patient's healthcare protocol. The technologies like kHealth are extremely useful especially during a pandemic when the in-person patient visits shifts to telemedicine appointments [7]. The clinicians can use kHealth framework during the telemedicine appointment to visually explores the PGHD along with the EMRs to better understand the patient's disease prognosis and suggest diagnoses. Also, a patient can use the kHealth framework to continuously monitor, appraise, and manage her chronic disease [8]. A detailed scenario for a pediatric asthma patient is given in [8, 9] [See Multimedia Appendix A].

The data collected from the kHealth framework is used to simulate Personalized Scores, and Digital Phenotype Score (DPS) which is a clinical equivalent for the Asthma Control Test (ACT) score. The DPS is used to categorize the asthma patients into their asthma control levels and recommend intervention strategies to the clinicians.

The chapter is divided into seven sections, Section 1 is introduction, Section 2 provides a brief overview of the kHealth framework and it's components, Section 3 explains the study methods, study design, and study protocol, Section 4 discusses the personalized scores followed by Section 5 on Digital Phenotype Score, Section 6 discusses actionable insights and causal intervention, and Section 7 concludes the chapter.

2. kHealth: knowledge-enabled healthcare

A knowledge-enabled healthcare framework, kHealth (**Figure 1**, Multimedia Appendix B), is a personalized framework for self monitoring of patient's symptoms, medication adherence, lung function, activity, etc. for pediatric asthma patients. The framework utilizes the existing medical knowledge along with the PGHD to assist the child, parent, and the clinician in better monitoring and

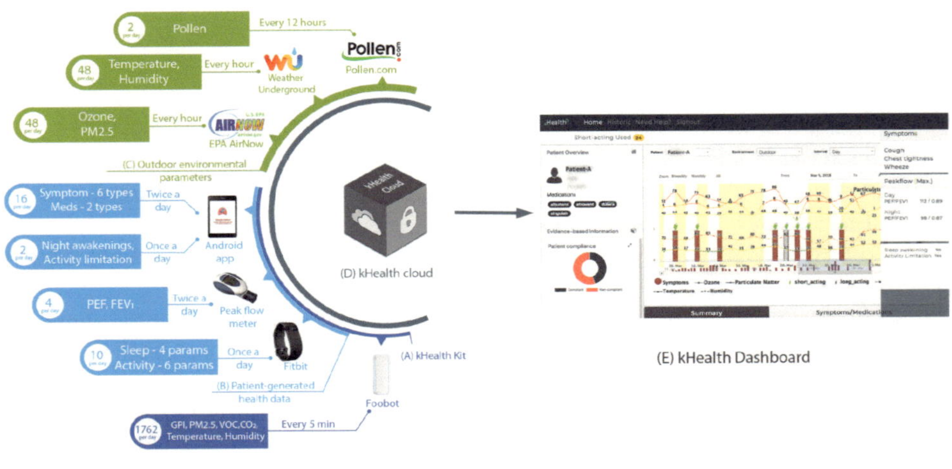

Figure 1.
kHealth architecture.

management of asthma. It provides an alternative to the traditional episodic clinician-centric health care by supporting real-time monitoring of a child's health condition. kHealth gathers empirical evidences to analyze and monitor disease progression and help in asthma management. It is a step towards exploring issues such as: What is the asthma control level of the child?, What is the medication compliance of the child?, What are the possible triggers for the child's asthma symptoms?, Can we understand the causal relationship between symptoms and possible triggers or factors responsible for the symptoms?, Can we predict asthma attacks based on the past data collected from the child?, etc. The kHealth framework consists of kHealth kit, kHealth cloud, and kHealth dashboard (described below).

2.1 kHealth kit

The kHealth kit consists of an android application (kHealth application) and a set of sensors (Foobot, Fitbit, and a Microlife Peak Flow Meter). Sections below provide a description of all the sensors and the type of data collected from them. kHealth framework uses the active and passive sensing techniques for data collection. Active sensing refers to the data collection where the child (or the parent) has to actively interact with the technology (e.g., answering questions in the kHealth application) [10]. Passive sensing refers to the data collected without active human interaction with the technology (e.g., Wearing Fitbit which automatically collects activity and sleep data) [10].

2.1.1 kHealth application

The kHealth application is built using the widely used Android platform. The application is designed in consultation with the clinician, tested with patients, and iteratively refined before reaching the current version used in the study [11]. The application asks questions similar to the ACT questionnaire (**Table 1**). The application captures symptoms, medication intake, and activity limitation because of asthma symptoms and nighttime awakenings using a questionnaire that the child is expected to answer twice a day. The application is personalized for every child,

kHealth application questions	Multiple-choice options
Are you currently experiencing any of the asthma-related symptoms below?	Cough, wheeze, chest tightness, hard and fast breathing, nose opens wide, cannot talk in full sentences, others
How many times did you take albuterol inhaler today because of asthma symptoms?	1, 2, 3, 4, 5, 6+
Have you had a wheeze, chest tightness, or asthma-related cough today?	Yes, No
How much did asthma or asthma symptoms limit your activity today?	None, a little, most of the day, at least half of the day
Did you take albuterol last night because of a cough or wheeze?	Yes, No
Did you wake up with a cough or wheeze last night?	Yes, No
Rescue medication question. For example, did you take albuterol today?	Yes, No
Controller medication question. For example, did you take Dulera today?	Yes, No

Table 1.
kHealth application questionnaire.

such as the medication (rescue and controller) information for every child is taken from the Electronic Medical Records (EMRs), and the medication intake questions are asked for the prescribed medications only. **Table 1** below shows the kHealth application questionnaire.

2.1.2 Fitbit

Fitbit is a wearable sensor which collects activity signals such daily step count, distance walked, floor climbed, sedentary minutes, lightly active minutes, fairly active minutes, very active minutes, and calories burned during the activities. The sleep signals includes minutes asleep at night, minutes awake, number of time the child woke up at night (number of awakenings), time spend in bed, minutes of REM (Rapid Eye Movement) sleep, minutes of light sleep, and minutes of deep sleep. The child is required to wear the Fitbit provided as part of the kHealth kit during the day and night.

2.1.3 Foobot

Foobot, is an indoor air quality sensor [12]. It is setup in the child's room or in the place in the house where the child spends majority of his/her time indoor. It connects to the home wifi, and records signal every 5-15 mins. The foobot records indoor temperature, humidity, carbon dioxide, volatile organic compound (VOC), and particulate matter 2.5 (PM2.5). The sensor turns red from green (healthy air quality) as an indicator of bad or unhealthy indoor air quality.

2.1.4 Microlife peak flow meter

Microlife Peak Flow Meter is used to record the child's lung function measures such as forced exhaled volume in 1 sec (FEV1) and peak expiratory flow (PEF). The peak flow meter has in-built memory to save upto 240 readings. Microlife has a free software available to the user to download their readings from the meter. The reading is taken by standing/sitting up straight, and blowing hard in the meter thrice. The device saves the highest of the three readings. As a backup, the child is also asked to input the reading in the kHealth application.

2.2 kHealth cloud

The data collected from the kHealth kit are synced in real time with Firebase, a Google cloud storage. Firebase provides active data listening for the client-side, which offers data persistence over a network failure and resyncs to the cloud when the network is restored. The kHealth application uses SQLite as the primary data storage and Firebase as the secondary data storage. Data from Firebase are available to Kno.e.sis researchers and clinicians for real-time analysis. Firebase provides a set of real-time database rules and user authentication that allow data access control on a per-user basis. It is built on the Google Cloud Platform, sharing the same level of data security [13].

2.3 kHealth Dashboard

kHealth Dashboard (**Figure 2**, Multimedia Appendix C) is a cloud-based platform that integrates and visualizes multi-modal PGHD data from the kHealth kit. kHealth Dashboard visually explores the correlations between the child's readings about their asthma symptoms, lung function, medication usage, and

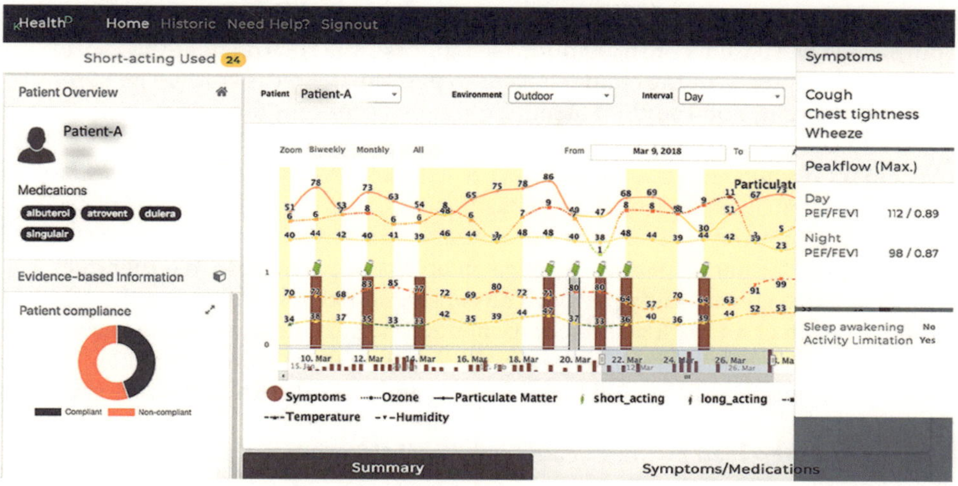

Figure 2.
kHealth dashboard.

environmental data [14]. In the **Figure 2**, the patient in consideration is prescribed Albuterol, Atrovent, Singulair and Dulera by the clinician, had 24 intakes of rescue medication (short-acting) during the course of the study, had symptoms of cough, chest tightness and wheeze, had activity limitations, and had maximum PEF/FEV1 values of 112/0.89 and 98/0.87 in the day and night respectively during the course of the study. The patient took rescue medications on 10th March when the outdoor environment condition was: ozone 44 (good), pollen 6 (medium), and particulate matter 78 (moderate). The next section describes the study procedure such as study design, study recruitment, etc.

3. Methods

The section describes the kHealth study design and study recruitment process.

3.1 Study design

kHealth is an observational longitudinal study involving collaboration among researchers from the Artificial Intelligence Institute at the University of South Carolina, Kno.e.sis—an Ohio Center of Excellence for BioHealth Innovations at Wright State University, and Dayton Children's Hospital (DCH), the latter consisting of a clinician and a nurse coordinator. The study was approved by the DCH institutional review board (IRB). The study uses off the shelf sensors and widely used technologies. The study comprises of 30 kits which allows parallel participation of up to 30 children at a time. The kHealth framework does not save any patient identified information such as name, date of birth, etc. The kHealth participant is given a kHealth ID such as KH001, KH002 to anonymize the data. The information to anonymize and de-anonymize is stored only at the DCH and is not shared with the researchers [15]. The information never leave the DCH servers.

3.2 Study recruitment

The study participants were recruited from Dayton Children's Hospital (DCH) under the guidance of a pediatric pulmonologist. The participants were children within the age group of 5-17 years diagnosed with asthma. The study coordinator approached the parents of the children seeking asthma treatment at the DCH. The parent, along with the child, consent to participate in the study. The parent provides consent, and the child assent by signing a consent form to participate in the study and giving permission to obtain the medical details from the EMRs. The participant recruitment was random, with asthma diagnoses as the only prerequisite. The type of asthma, such as persistent, non persistent, exercise induced, and non exercise-induced asthma was not taken into consideration for the study recruitment. The participant were given an option to participate in either one month or three month study period. The consented participant were given a brief demonstration of all the kHealth components. The participants also had access to a user guide, tutorial video in the application to make it more accessible. The contact information of the study coordinator, and the kHealth team were saved in the user guide to reach out in case of any technical difficulties. The technical difficulties were resolved by the kHealth team while keeping the participant identity anonymized.

The PGHD collected from the pediatric patients using the kHealth framework is used to generate personalized insights into one's healthcare protocol. The next section describes the personalization in chronic diseases like asthma and how does the PGHD can be used for better disease management, and self appraisal.

4. Personalization

Asthma is a personalized disease. An asthma patient differs from another patient with respect to their asthma symptoms, possible triggers, medication adherence, and asthma control levels. The below observation comes from preliminary analysis and anecdotal evidence from the data. For example, Patients A and B, both in the same asthma control, and severity level category and have fall pollen allergies. However, Patient A does not show symptoms until the pollen crosses the threshold 6 (pollen: medium [16]) whereas Patient B starts showing symptoms as soon as the pollen levels goes beyond 3 (pollen: low-medium [16]). Personalization in the kHealth framework is able to capture these granularities (symptoms, medication intake, difficulty sleeping and reduced activity due to the outdoor environmental conditions) at a given point in time. We also observe patients in one asthma control level category are more proactive towards their health and medication adherence resulting into fewer We define personalized scores such as Symptom Score, Medication (Rescue, Controller) compliance Scores, Activity Score, etc. to get a real time insight into the patient's health condition unlike the irregular ACT administered during the clinic visits. The personalized scores helps in real time categorization of the patient into their asthma control levels.

4.1 Symptom score

Symptom score for a child is defined by the number of symptoms experienced by the child during the course of deployment period. The symptom severity (Chest Tightness being more severe than wheeze and cough, etc) is ignored for the symptom score estimation.

$$SS = \frac{Total\, symptoms\ experienced\ by\ the\, child}{Study\, Period} \tag{1}$$

4.2 Activity score

Activity Score of a child is the number of days the child had restricted activity during the study duration. The kHealth application asks a multiple-choice question: How much did asthma symptoms limit your activity today? with four options: none, a little, half of the day, and most of the day. The options are weighted on a scale of 0-3, respectively.

$$AcS = \frac{Number\ of\ days\ of\ activity\ restriction\left(weighted\ option\right)}{Study\ Period} \tag{2}$$

4.3 Awakening score

The Awakening Score (AwS) is the measure of number of nights the child woke up because of asthma symptoms during the study period. The kHealth application asks a multiple-choice question: Did you wake up with wheeze, cough, or any asthma-related symptoms?

$$AwS = \frac{Number\ of\ days\ child\ woke\ up\ due\ to\ asthma}{Study\ Period} \tag{3}$$

4.4 Rescue compliance score

The kHealth application collects data on the intake of the rescue medication (short-acting bronchodilators) by asking questions such as Did you take albuterol today? Rescue Compliance Score (RCS) is defined as the number of times the child took the rescue medication during the study period. The rescue medication is taken to mitigate or prevent the symptoms.

$$RCS = \frac{Total\ Resuce\ medication\ intake\ by\ the\ child}{Study\ Period} \tag{4}$$

4.5 Controller compliance score

The kHealth application asks questions (eg, Did you take Dulera today?) about the intake of the controller medication (long-term control medication). An asthmatic patient is prescribed a controller medication, which is supposed to take at least once a day depending on the asthma control levels. The Controller Compliance Score (CCS) is defined as the fraction of the number of days the child took the controller medication during the study period.

$$CCS = \frac{Total\ Controller\ medication\ intake\ by\ the\ child}{Study\ Period} \tag{5}$$

The threshold for Controller Compliance Score is defined as Highly Compliant for score greater than and equal to 0.70, Well Compliant for score greater than and equal to 0.30 and less than 0.70, and Poorly Compliant for score less than 0.30.

Let us take an example scenario to better understand the personalized scores and generate actionable insights into their asthma management. Alice is ten yrs. old and clinically (using the ACT score) categorized into Not Well Controlled asthma control level. She and her parents agreed to participate in the one month kHealth study period. According to the data collected using the kHealth framework, Alice had ten incidents of cough, ten incidents of wheeze, five chest tightness, no incidents of hard and fast breathing, and no incidents of cannot talk in full sentences. She woke up during the night due to asthma symptoms on ten nights and had asthma symptom related activity limitation for five days. She had her controller medication for twenty days and had five rescue medication during her study period. Alice had a Symptom Score of 0.83 (=25/30; 10 cough +10 wheeze +5 chest tightness = 25 symptoms), Awakening Score of 0.33 (=10/33), Activity Score of 0.16 (=5/30), Rescue Compliance Score of 0.16 (=5/30), and Controller Compliance Score of 0.66 (=20/30). Alice is Well Compliant for her controller medications. The next section utilizes the above personalized scores for real time categorization of the child into their asthma control levels.

5. Digital phenotype score: Asthma categorization

The child (or the parent) is given an Asthma Control Test (ACT) at the regular checkup appointment. The ACT asks questions about the asthma symptoms, school days missed, night time awakenings, inhaler intakes etc. in the past four weeks. The child is categorized into one of the three asthma control levels of Well Controlled, Not Well Controlled, and Very Poorly Controlled asthma based on the scores obtained in the test. The ACT is used to analyze the asthma management of the child in between the visits, and also as a measure of Does the therapy helps the child's asthma management?, or Is there a need for intervention and change in therapy/treatment protocol? The ACT is administered during the infrequent clinic visit and asks questions about past four weeks, it is highly unlikely the child or the parent will remember all the relevant asthma episodes which leads to incorrect asthma control level classification [17, 18].

Digital Phenotype Score (DPS) defined using the kHealth data and National Heart, Lung, and Blood Institute (NHLBI) guidelines to categorize the child into their asthma control level overcomes the limitations of the ACT scores [19–22]. The child/parent and the clinician do not have to wait for the clinic visits to get an analysis of the current asthma management of the child. The clinician can use the DPS for early and timely intervention to recognize any barriers to the current therapy. The DPS is a quantified measure of the symptom score, activity score, awakening score, and rescue compliance score. The DPS of greater than and equal to one is classified as Very Poorly Controlled asthma, greater than equal to 0.28 and less than one is classified as Not Well Controlled asthma, and less than 0.28 is classified as Well Controlled asthma. In the case of Alice, the DPS is 1.48 (=0.83 + 0.16 + 0.33 + 0.16). According to the thresholds defined her asthma is classified as Very Poorly Controlled.

6. Causal intervention and actionable insights

The Personalized scores along with Digital Phenotype Score related categorization can be used to generate actionable insights into a patient's healthcare protocol [21, 23]. These insights in future can also be used by the clinician to design a perfect intervention strategies/policies (**Figure 3**) for better health outcome and improving the quality of life of the patient [24, 25]. Let us take an example scenario, A child categorized as having Very Poorly Controlled asthma using the DPS, suffering with

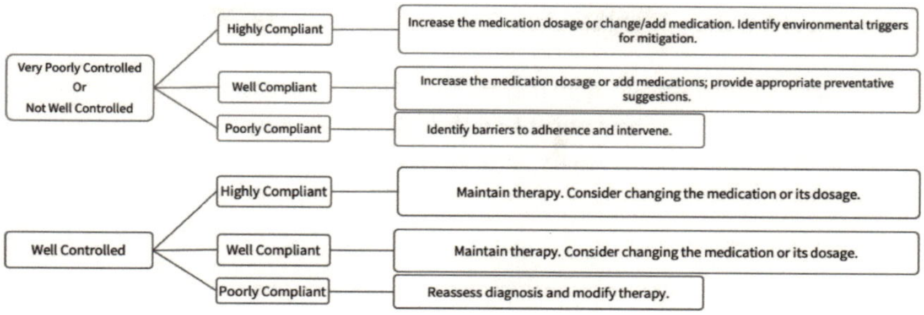

Figure 3.
Root cause analysis techniques can be used to access the path specific policy update for intervention strategies.

a high symptom score and Highly Compliant for the controller medication. The CCS and the DPS sheds light on an important aspect of the child's asthma management that although the child is highly compliant towards the controller medication but still suffers from high symptom score. This is an opportunity for the clinician to intervene with either increasing the medication dosage, or change or add a medication, and identify the environment triggers for mitigation. On the other hand a child with Very Poorly Controlled asthma and poorly compliant with the controller medication is in the worst health condition and requires immediate attention from the clinician and support from the parent/caregiver. The intervention strategy would be to identify the barriers to medication adherence and suggest mitigation/alternative efforts. A child with well controlled asthma and highly compliant with the medication is a use case when the child/parent are proactive towards the asthma management. In this scenario the clinician can choose to intervene with either maintaining the therapy or considering changing the medication or lowering the dosage.

In the case of Alice, she is well compliant with her controller medication and as per the DPS has very poorly controlled asthma. The clinician can intervene in her asthma management protocol with either increasing the medication dosage or adding a new medication since her current medications are unable to control her asthma, and also provide appropriate preventive suggestions to reduce future asthma exacerbation.

7. Conclusions

The digital healthcare technologies such as IoTs, self-reporting applications, wearables can be used to improve the quality of life of the pediatric asthma patients. The kHealth framework has moved the current healthcare approach from clinician-centric to patient-centric. The child/parent feels empowered to take control of their health management. The clinician can include the framework like kHealth in their current protocol which is especially useful during the pandemic when the care has shifted from in-person clinic visit to tele-medicine appointment. The asthma patients are prescribed Longacting combination inhalers, Long-acting inhaled steroids or Oral Steroids depending on how controlled is a patient's asthma condition. The long term use of steroids leads to a growth suppression, adrenal gland suppression, osteoporosis, increase a risk of high blood pressure, heart attack, increase in appetite leading to weight gain and eventually increase in body mass index [26]. The early and timely intervention strategies discussed can be used to avoid overuse of the steroid medications, and can eliminate the vicious cycle of asthma affecting obesity or obesity affects asthma.

Acknowledgements

This research is supported by National Institutes of Health under the Grant Number 1 R01HD087132. The content of this study is solely the responsibility of the authors and does not necessarily represent the official views of the National Institutes of Health.

Conflict of interest

The authors declare no conflict of interest.

Abbreviations

PGHD	Patient Generated Health Data
IoTs	Internet of Things
DCH	Dayton Children's Hospital
ACT	Asthma Control Test
DPS	Digital Phenotype Score
IRB	Institutional Revenue Board
EMR	Electronic Medical Record
NHLBI	National Heart, Lung, and Blood Institute
CT	Chest Tightness
HFB	Hard and Fast Breathing
CTFS	Cannot talk in full sentences
PM2.5	Particulate Matter 2.5
VOC	Volatile Organic Compounds
SS	Symptom Score
AcS	Activity Score
AwS	Awakening Score
RCS	Rescue Compliance Score
CCS	Controller Compliance Score

Multimedia Appendix A

Augmented health with personalized data and AI, TEDx2020, The University of South Carolina, Oct 21, 2020, Accessible at: https://bit.ly/3ahJEhy

Multimedia Appendix B

The kHealth project webpage: https://bit.ly/3aX4Ng0

Multimedia Appendix C

kHealth Dashboard video: https://bit.ly/2ZfeSj8

Author details

Utkarshani Jaimini[1,2*] and Amit Sheth[1,2]

1 Artificial Intelligence Institute, Columbia, SC, USA

2 University of South Carolina, Columbia, SC, USA

*Address all correspondence to: ujaimini@email.sc.edu

References

[1] Boulet, L.P., Boulay, M.` E., Chanez, Humbert, Bateman, Soriano, Gershon, van Manen, Cazzola, Settipane and Guerra, 2011. Asthma-related comorbidities. Expert review of respiratory medicine, 5(3), pp.377-393.

[2] Jaimini U. CDC. 2018. Asthma Surveillance Data. https://www.cdc.gov/asthma/asthmadata.htm [Accessed: 19 January 2021]

[3] van den Bemt, L., Kooijman, S., Linssen, V., Lucassen, P., Muris, J., Slabbers, G. and Schermer, T., 2010. How does asthma influence the daily life of children? Results of focus group interviews. Health and quality of life outcomes, 8(1), pp.1-10.

[4] Med.stanford.edu. 2021. https://med.stanford.edu/content/dam/sm/cerc/documents/SCC MTM Asthma%20 Management%20Protocol.pdf [Accessed 10 February 2021].

[5] Sheth, A., 2014, March. Transforming big data into smart data: Deriving value via harnessing volume, variety, and velocity using semantic techniques and technologies. In 2014 IEEE 30th International Conference on Data Engineering (ICDE) (pp. 2-2). IEEE Computer Society.

[6] Choe, E.K., Lee, B., Andersen, T.O., Wilcox, L. and Fitzpatrick, G., 2018. Harnessing the power of patient-generated data. IEEE Pervasive Computing, 17(2), pp.50-56.

[7] Hodgkins, M., Barron, M., Jevaji, S. and Lloyd, S., 2021. Physician requirements for adoption of telehealth following the SARS-CoV-2 pandemic. npj Digital Medicine, 4(1), pp.1-3.

[8] Sheth, A., Jaimini, U. and Yip, H.Y., 2018. How will the internet of things enable augmented personalized health?. IEEE intelligent systems, 33(1), pp.89-97.

[9] Sheth, A., Jaimini, U., Thirunarayan, K. and Banerjee, T., 2017, September. Augmented personalized health: how smart data with IoTs and AI is about to change healthcare. In 2017 IEEE 3rd International Forum on Research and Technologies for Society and Industry (RTSI) (pp. 1-6). IEEE.

[10] Sheth, A., Anantharam, P. and Thirunarayan, K., 2014. khealth: Proactive personalized actionable information for better healthcare. In Workshop Personal Data Analytics in the Internet of Things.

[11] Tinschert, P., Jakob, R., Barata, F., Kramer, J.N. and Kowatsch, T., 2017. The potential of mobile apps for improving asthma self-management: a review of publicly available and well-adopted asthma apps. JMIR mHealth and uHealth, 5(8), p.e113.

[12] Jaimini, U., Banerjee, T., Romine, W., Thirunarayan, K., Sheth, A. and Kalra, M., 2017. Investigation of an indoor air quality sensor for asthma management in children. IEEE sensors letters, 1(2), pp.1-4.

[13] Jaimini U. Cloud.google. 2018. https://cloud.google.com/security/compliance/[Accessed: 12 February 2021]

[14] Sridharan, V., 2018. Sensor Data Streams Correlation Platform for Asthma Management.

[15] Sharma, S., Chen, K. and Sheth, A., 2018. Toward practical privacy-preserving analytics for IoT and cloud-based healthcare systems. IEEE Internet Computing, 22(2), pp.42-51.

[16] Pollen.com https://www.pollen.com/ [Accessed: 20 February 2021]

[17] Bime, C., Gerald, J.K., Wei, C.Y., Holbrook, J.T., Teague, W.G., Wise, R.A. and Gerald, L.B., 2016. Measurement

characteristics of the childhood Asthma-Control Test and a shortened, child-only version. NPJ primary care respiratory medicine, 26(1), pp.1-7.

[18] Carroll, W., 2013. Limitations of asthma control questionnaires in the management and follow up of childhood asthma. Paediatric respiratory reviews, 14(4), pp.229-231.

[19] Jain, S.H., Powers, B.W., Hawkins, J.B. and Brownstein, J.S., 2015. The digital phenotype. Nature biotechnology, 33(5), pp.462-463.

[20] Merchant, R., Inamdar, R., Henderson, K., Barrett, M., Su, J.G., Riley, J., Van Sickle, D. and Stempel, D., 2018. Digital health intervention for asthma: patient-reported value and usability. JMIR mHealth and uHealth, 6(6), p.e133.

[21] Jaimini, U., Thirunarayan, K., Kalra, M., Venkataraman, R., Kadariya, D. and Sheth, A., 2018. "How Is My Child's Asthma?" digital phenotype and actionable insights for pediatric asthma. JMIR pediatrics and parenting, 1(2), p.e11988.

[22] Cloutier, M.M., Baptist, A.P., Blake, K.V., Brooks, E.G., Bryant-Stephens, T., DiMango, E., Dixon, A.E., Elward, K.S., Hartert, T., Krishnan, J.A. and Ouellette, D.R., 2020. 2020 Focused Updates to the Asthma Management Guidelines: A Report from the National Asthma Education and Prevention Program Coordinating Committee Expert Panel Working Group. Journal of Allergy and Clinical Immunology, 146(6), pp.1217-1270.

[23] Birnbaum, F., Lewis, D.M., Rosen, R. and Ranney, M.L., 2015. Patient engagement and the design of digital health. Academic emergency medicine: official journal of the Society for Academic Emergency Medicine, 22(6), p.754.

[24] Prosperi, M., Guo, Y., Sperrin, M., Koopman, J.S., Min, J.S., He, X., Rich, S., Wang, M., Buchan, I.E. and Bian, J., 2020. Causal inference and counterfactual prediction in machine learning for actionable healthcare. Nature Machine Intelligence, 2(7), pp.369-375.

[25] Gaveikaite, V., Grundstrom, C., Lourida, K., Winter, S., Priori, R., Chouvarda, I. and Maglaveras, N., 2020. Developing a strategic understanding of telehealth service adoption for COPD care management: A causal loop analysis of healthcare professionals. PloS one, 15(3), p.e0229619.

[26] Nhsinform.scot. 2021. Corticosteroids. [online] https://www.nhsinform.scot/tests-and-treatments/medicines-and-medical-aids/types-of-medicine/corticosteroids [Accessed 23 February 2021].

Chapter 4

Epigenetic Regulation of Th2 Response in Asthma by Non-Coding RNAs

Yanhua Niu, Chao Wang, Xiaoyan Dong and Nanbert Zhong

Abstract

Asthma is a common chronic inflammatory disease. Pathogenic mechanism underlying asthma is complex. The inflammatory response of asthma includes lymphocytes (T, B cells), ILC2, eosinophils and other types of immune and inflammatory cells. T CD4+ T helper 2 cells (Th2 cells) are thought to play a central role in regulating the phenotype of allergic asthma. Asthma is often closely associated with Th1/Th2 cell imbalance. Non-coding RNAs (ncRNAs) are non-protein coding RNA molecules in the transcriptome, mainly including microRNAs (miRNAs), long non-coding RNAs and circRNAs, etc., which are widely found in eukaryotic transcriptome and participate in the regulation of a variety of biological processes. ncRNAs are considered to function as modulators of the immune system. Their biological changes represent an important mechanism for the development of immune-mediated diseases. This chapter mainly discusses the epigenetic regulation of Th2 cells and their cytokines in asthma by non-coding RNAs. It helps us to better understand the pathogenesis of asthma and find potential asthma biomarkers.

Keywords: asthma, Th2, cytokines, non-coding RNAs

1. Introduction

Asthma is a chronic airway inflammatory disease, associated with variable expiratory airflow limitation, clinically manifested as recurrent wheezing, shortness of breath, chest tightness, cough and other symptoms [1]. It has affected more than 300 million people worldwide and has become a major public health concern [2].

Non-coding RNAs (ncRNAs) are a class of non-coding RNA molecules widely found in eukaryotes and involved in a variety of biological regulatory processes. They have been extensively studied in human diseases [3–5]. NcRNAs mainly includes microRNAs (miRNAs), long non-coding RNAs (lncRNAs), circular RNAs (circRNAs), etc.

The pathogenesis of asthma remains extremely complicated and the detailed mechanisms are not clarified. The most common phenotype is eosinophilic inflammation associated with Th2 response and concomitant atopic diseases. Asthma is often closely associated with Th1/Th2 cell imbalance. Th2 cells secrete Th2 cytokines, including interleukin-IL-4, IL-5, and IL-13, which amplify type 2 inflammation, while Th1 cells secrete Th1 cytokines [interferon IFN-γ, IL-2, lymphoid (LT)-α, and tumor necrosis factor TNF-α, which limit type 2 inflammation [6, 7].

The CD^{4+} T cells are major effector cells driving asthma-related inflammation and the skewing of T cells into Th2 cells can lead to imbalance of Th1-type and Th2-type cytokines, which promotes the onset and progression of asthma [8, 9]. Understanding the factors contributing to Th2 in asthma will provide important insights into the underlying pathogenesis of the disease. The skewing of T cells into Th2 cells causes an imbalance of Th1-type and Th2-type cytokines, which promotes the onset and progression of asthma. A number of studies have shown that ncRNAs may play an important role in Th2 cell-mediated inflammation in asthma. This chapter mainly discusses the epigenetic regulation of Th2 response in asthma by non-coding RNAs, in order to better understand the disease pathogenesis and find potential asthma biomarkers.

2. Regulation of microRNAs on Th2 in asthma

MicroRNAs are a group of small nonprotein-coding RNAs that are 18–25 nucleotides in length. They act as transcriptional regulators involved in many complex human disorders and in biological processes including cell proliferation and apoptosis [10–12]. MiRNA expression profiles have also been described in some allergic conditions and asthma [13]. Previous studies have suggested that miRNAs are involved in the development of allergic diseases by affecting Th1/Th2 polarization, promoting chronic inflammation and tissue remodeling of epithelial cells, and activating innate immune cells [13]. Th2-mediated inflammation is the core of the pathogenesis of allergic asthma. Th2-dominated T lymphocytes regulate allergic diseases by secreting a variety of proinflammatory cytokines. Recent studies have shown that most of the miRNAs involved increase Th2 cytokine secretion, reduce Th1 cytokine secretion, promote T cell differentiation to Th2, or play a role in the proliferation and hypertrophy of bronchial smooth muscle cells [14–16]. There is no doubt that miRNA plays a role in the regulation of asthma inflammation. MiRNAs may regulate Th2 in asthma by affecting Th1/Th2 balance, secretion of Th2 cytokines and related signaling pathways.

2.1 Regulation of Th2 cytokines by miRNAs

Th2-mediated inflammation is the core of the pathogenesis of allergic asthma. Typical cytokines involved in the Th2 response are IL-4, IL-5, and IL-13. Pua et al. [15] studied the miRNA related to Th2 cell differentiation and cytokine production by combining experimental and bioinformatics methods, and found that both miR-24 and miR-27 inhibited the production of IL-4 in T cells in vitro. Inhibition of the function of miR-145 suppresses house dust mites (HDM)-induced mucus hypersecretion in airway epithelial cells, eosinophilic inflammation, th2 cytokine production, and airway hyperresponsiveness as effectively as dexamethasone treatment. This study shows that miR-145 plays a key role in the occurrence and pathogenesis of allergic airway disease caused by house dust mites by inducing the release of IL-5 and IL-13 from Th2 cells [14]. Panganiban et al. found a variety of differentially expressed miRNAs in the serum of patients with asthma, and predicted that these miRNAs could regulate IL-5 and other TH2 mediators [17]. It was further confirmed that IL-5 was regulated by miRNA, and miR-1248 was identified as a positive regulator of IL-5 expression [17]. IL-10 levels are reduced in asthmatic patients, and the relative deficiency of IL-10 allows continued production of allergenic cytokines, such as IL-4 and IL-5, and other pro-inflammatory cytokines, including IL-1, TNF-α, and IL-6 [18]. Inhibition of miR-106a promotes IL-10 secretion and helps alleviate asthma symptoms by increasing Th2 response in a mouse model of asthma [19]. Simpson et al. demonstrated that the miR-17 ~ 92 cluster, and specifically miR-19a, promotes Th2 cytokine production by simultaneously targeting inhibitors of the NF-κB, JAK–STAT, and PI (3)K pathways. Their data also suggest that upregulation of miR-19a in asthma airway T cells may be an indicator and cause of increased IL-13 production and may contribute to type 2 inflammation in asthma [20]. In ovalbumin (OVA)-induced asthma mice, miR-146a significantly inhibited inflammatory cell infiltration in bronchoalveolar lavage fluid (BALF) and reduced levels of OVA-specific IgE and T-helper 2 cell type cytokines (IL-5 and IL-13) [21]. MiR-146a may act as a novel therapeutic molecule to modulate the immune response of asthma. MiR-155 has been shown to be a key modulator of the immune system. MiR-155 may regulate Th2 inflammation by regulating Th2 cell differentiation and the secretion of IL-4, IL-5 and IL-13. These studies suggest that targeting miR-155 may be a novel therapeutic strategy for human diseases induced by the Th2 immune response, such as asthma [22, 23]. It has been found that let-7 microRNAs inhibit IL-13 expression and thereby modulate Th 2 inflammation in an IL-13-dependent mouse model of allergic airway inflammation [24]. In ovalbumin (OVA) -induced asthma mice, intranasal administration of miR-410 significantly reduced the expression of IL-4 and IL-13 and effectively inhibited airway inflammation in OVA-induced asthmatic mice. Therefore, targeting to increase the expression of miR-410 may be a promising approach for the treatment of allergic asthma [25]. In a mouse model of asthma induced by ovalbumin, the researchers tested the airway hyperresponsiveness, rt-pcr detection of miR - 135 a content in the lung tissue of mice, HE staining to evaluate the pathological changes of lung tissue and ELISA and immunohistochemical detection of bronchoalveolar lavage fluid (BALF) and lung tissue of the tumor necrosis factor (TNF) - alpha, interleukin (IL) - 6, IL - 5 and eosinophils chemokine expression. The results of this study showed that miR-135a decreased expression in asthmatic mice, and miR-135a reduced the levels of inflammatory cytokines TNF-α, IL-6, IL-5 and eosinophilic chemokines in the lung tissue of mice, thereby reducing airway inflammation. Further research in this study showed that miR-135a inhibited airway inflammation in asthmatic mice by regulating the JAK/STAT signaling pathway [26]. Previous studies in human, animal models, and cell culture have shown that the Th2 cytokine IL-13 is an important cause of airway epithelial abnormalities in asthma [27–29]. Kuperman et al. used miRNA microarray to analyze the bronchial epithelial cells of asthmatic patients and healthy control subjects, and found that the expression of miR-34/449 family members was decreased in asthmatic patients. IL-13-induced reduction of miR-34/449 in bronchial epithelial cells may lead to changes in epithelial differentiation common in asthma [30]. Zhang et al. investigated the role of miR-221-3p in airway eosinophilic inflammation in a mouse model of HDM-induced allergic airway inflammation, and showed that epithelial miR-221-3p expression was reduced in asthma. Airway overexpression of miR-221-3p induced the expression of IL-4, IL-5, and IL-13 mRNAs in the lungs of mice induced by HDM [31]. The expression of miR-26a, miR-146a, and miR-31 and cytokine levels of IL-5, IL-8, IL-12, and TNF-α were measured in lung tissue and bronchoalveolar lavage fluid of asthmatic mice and children with ovalbumin induced asthma. The results showed that miR-26a, miR-146a, and miR-31 were significantly elevated in asthma, and were involved in the progression of asthma by regulating the expression of inflammatory cytokines IL-5, IL-8, IL-12, and TNF-α [32]. The systems immunology approach (the Impact of Differential Expression Across Layers, a network-based algorithm to prioritize disease-relevant miRs based on the central role of their targets in the molecular interactome) was used to antagonize miRs (miR27b, miR206, miR106b, miR203, and miR23b) in vitro, which has significantly reduced cytokine production in Th2 cells. These results suggest that these miRNAs play an important role in the

Th2-driven immune response [33]. In conclusion, many miRNAs play an important role in asthma by regulating the secretion of Th2 cytokines. They may be new targets for the treatment of asthma in the future.

2.2 Regulation of Th1/Th2 balance by miRNAs

Qui et al. detected the levels of Th1- and Th2-related cytokines by ELISA, performed microRNA microarray assay and analyzed the differentiation marker gene of T helper cells by qRT-PCR. The results indicated that an imbalance of Th1/Th2 cells was present in the asthmatic patients; Runx3 expression is decreased in asthmatic patients; overexpression of Runx3 could restore the Th1/Th2 balance; miR-371, miR-138, miR-544, miR-145, and miR-214 could directly bind to the 3'-UTR of Runx3. All these findings suggest that these miRNAs may be involved in Th1/Th2 imbalance in asthma by regulating Runx3 [34]. One study used predictive algorithms dentified potential direct miR-21 targets among IL-13-regulated lung transcripts such as IL-12p35 mRNA that was decreased in IL-13 transgenic mice. MiR-21 was significantly elevated in ovalbumin-induced mice lungs, suggesting that miR-21 regulates Th1 to Th2 phenotypic transformation by decreasing the mouse IL-12p35 transcriptome [16]. Reduced levels of miR-29b were found in the lungs and spleens of OVA-induced asthmatic mice, and this miRNA indirectly affects the Th2 response by regulating the production of T-box transcription factors and IFN-γ in T helper cells [35]. Low expression of miR-29b in asthmatic lung can increase the production of IFN-γ and restore the balance of Th1/Th2 in asthmatic lung [36]. The researchers evaluated the relationship between miRNA levels in small extracellular vesicles (sEVs) from nasal washing and pulmonary function parameters in children with mild to moderate or severe asthma compared to healthy controls. The results showed that lower levels of miR-34a, miR-92b and miR-210 in children with sEVs in this study were associated with pulmonary function and airway obstruction. Subsequent functional pathway analysis showed reduced levels of miR-92b, miR-210, and miR-34a in epithelial-derived sEVs in asthma, and these miRNAs regulate Th2 polarization and dendritic cell maturation [37].

2.3 miRNAs regulation of Th2 differentiation via signaling pathways

Inhibition of microRNA-126 (miR-126) has been shown to effectively inhibit Th2-driven airway inflammation, mucus hypersecretion, and airway hyperresponsiveness in a model of ovalbumin (OVA) -induced chronic asthma [38]. The blocking of miR-126 leads to the enhanced expression of POU domain 2 related factor 1, which activates the transcription factor PU1, that changes the function of Th2 cells by negatively regulating the expression of GATA3 [39]. In childhood asthma, miRNA-451a was found to inhibit Th2 cell differentiation by down-regulating proto-oncogene 1 (ETS1). This study reveals that miRNA-451a-ETS1 axis dysfunction is a novel molecular mechanism that underlies the pathogenesis of childhood asthma [40]. A study has shown that miR-1165-3p targets IL-13 and PPM1A to control Th2 differentiation and pulmonary inflammation in asthma. miR-1165-3p inhibits the Th2 response of allergy through the STAT and AKT signaling pathways by targeted inhibition of protein phosphatase, Mg 2+/Mn 2+ – dependent 1A (PPM1A), thus proving that miR-1165-3p and PPM1A may be effective targets for the prevention and treatment of allergic asthma and related diseases [41]. The miR-29c/B7-H3 axis plays an important role in asthmatic children by regulating Th2/Th17 cell differentiation, and may provide a new target for asthma treatment [42]. The role of Th2-mediated microRNAs in asthma are summarized in the **Table 1** (**Figure 1**).

Altered MiRNA	Expressi-on pattern	Targets/ Regulators	Signaling Pathway	Function	Ref
miR-24 miR-27	Down-regulated	IL-4		limit IL-4 production	[15]
miR-145	Up-regulated	IL-5, IL-13		promote the production of Th2 cytokines	[14]
miR-1248	Up-regulated	IL-5		elevates Th2 cytokine levels.	[17]
miR-106a	Up-regulated	IL-10		regulate Th2 cytokine secretion	[19]
miR-17 ~ 92 cluster /miR-19a	Up-regulated	IL-13	NF-κB, JAK–STAT/ PI (3)K pathways	promotes Th2 cytokine production	[20]
miR-146a	Up-regulated	IL-5, IL-13		reduce the levels of IgE and T-helper 2 cytokines	[21]
miR-155	Up-regulated	IL-4, IL-5 IL-13		regulate Th2 cell differentiation and the secretion of IL-4, IL-5 and IL-13	[22, 23]
Let-7a	Down-regulated	IL-13		targeting IL-13 alleviates asthmatic phenotype	[24]
miR-410	Down-regulated	IL-4 IL-13		reduce the expression of IL-4 and IL-13	[25]
miR-135a	Down-regulated	TNF-α, IL-6, IL-5		Reduce airway inflammation	[26]
miR-34/449	Down-regulated	IL-13		Regulate differentiation of epithelial cells	[30]
miR-221-3p	Down-regulated	IL-4, IL-5, IL-13		correlate the type 2 status in asthma.	[31]
miR-26a, miR-146a, miR-31	Up-regulated	IL-5, IL-8, IL-12, TNF-α		Promote the expression of cytokines	[32]
mir27b, mir206, mir106b, mir203, mir23b				Reduce the production of cytokines in Th2 cells	[33]
miR-371, miR138, miR-544, miR-145 miR-214	Up-regulated	Runx3	—	regulates Th1/Th2 balance in asthma.	[34]
miR-21	Up-regulated	IL-12p35	IL-13Rα1, STAT6	regulates Th1 to Th2 phenotypic transformation	[16]
miR-29b	Down-regulated	T-box IFN-γ		regulate Th1 / Th2 balance in asthma	[35, 36]

Altered MiRNA	Expressi-on pattern	Targets/ Regulators	Signaling Pathway	Function	Ref
miR-92b, miR-210, miR-34a	Down-regulated			regulate Th2 polarization and dendritic cell maturation.	[37]
miR-29c	Up-regulated		miR-29c / B7-H3	regulate Th2/Th17 cell differentiation an	[42]
miR-126	Down-regulated			inhibit Th2-driven airway inflammation	[39]
miRNA-451a	Down-regulated	ETS1	miRNA-451a-ETS1	inhibit Th2 cell differentiation	[40]
miR-1165-3p	Down-regulated	IL-13 and PPM1A		Suppresses Th2 differentiation	[41]
miR-21 miR-19a				promoting differentiation of T cells towards Th2	[16, 43, 44]

Table 1.
Regulation of Th2 in asthma by miRNAs.

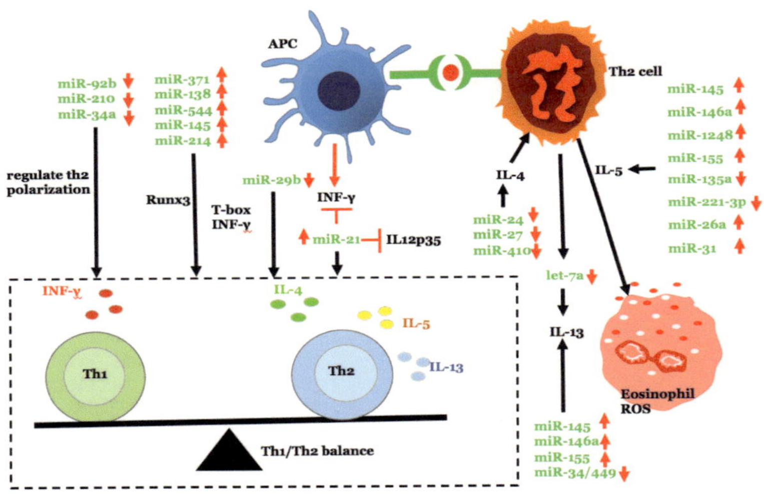

Figure 1.
Regulation of Th2 in asthma by miRNAs. Th1 and Th2 are in equilibrium. miR-34a, miR-92b and miR-210 regulate Th2 polarization. MiRNAs such as miR-371, miR-138, miR-544 and miR-145 affect Th1/Th2 balance of asthma by regulating Runx3. MiR-21 regulates Th1 and Th2 balance by regulating IL-12p35 transcripts. As shown in the figure, miR-24, miR-27, miR-410, let-7a, miR-145, miR-146a, miR-1248 and other miRNAs regulate the secretion of Th2 cytokines, such as IL-4, IL-5 and IL-13, through up-regulation or down-regulation in asthma, and affect the occurrence and development of asthma.

3. lncRNA regulate Th2 response in asthma

LncRNA refers to a class of RNA molecules with a length greater than 200 nucleotides which do not have the function of coding RNAs. LncRNAs are mainly involved in gene expression regulation at the transcription, post-transcription, translation and epigenetic levels, and are widely involved in various life processes such as cell proliferation, differentiation, apoptosis, migration, aging and metabolism [45, 46]. Abundant expressions of lncRNAs were found in T cell lineages, suggesting that these transcripts play important roles in T cell development and differentiation [47]. Studies have found that some lncRNAs play important roles in the pathogenesis of asthma by regulating Th1/Th2 balance and Th2 inflammatory response [3, 48]. Understanding how lncRNAs alter gene expression to promote Th2 skewing may provide new insights into mechanisms and therapeutic targets for asthma.

3.1 Regulation of Th1/Th2 balance by lncRNAs

The gene encoding lncRNA MALTA1, a highly conserved nuclear lncRNA, is located on chromosome 11 (11q13.1). MALTA1 is highly expressed in most cells [49]. Liang et al. [50] conducted a cohort study of 772 asthmatic patients and 441 healthy controls, and found that the expression of MALAT1 was up-regulated and the expression of miR-155 was down-regulated in the blood of asthmatic patients. MALAT1 expression was inversely associated with impaired lung function and the Th1 / Th2 ratio, suggesting that its role was to impairs lung function by promoting the Th2 response. That is, the up-regulated expression of MALAT1 can induce the production of Th2 cytokines and inhibit the release of Th1 cytokines. Further study of the experiment showed that MALAT1 sponging miR-155 could alter the Th1/Th2 balance within CD^{4+} T cells through cytotoxic T-lymphocyte antigen 4 (CTLA-4) dependent mechanism. This study highlights the novel role of lncRNA MALTA1 in the development of Th2 in asthma. Wei et al. found that lncRNA PVT1 expression was increased in ozone-induced mouse asthma models, and the lncRNA PVT1-miR-15a-5p axis promoted Th1/Th2 imbalance in CD4 + T cells by activating the PI3K-Akt- signaling pathway [51].

3.2 lncRNA regulate Th2-type inflammation in asthma

Zhu et al. assessed expression of lncRNAs in peripheral blood samples of patients with eosinophilic asthma, neutrophilic asthma and healthy controls using RNA-sequencing. In this study, it was found that the expression of LNC_000127 was increased in eosinophilic asthma, and knockdown of LNC_000127 (refer to this article for details) reduced the expression of CCR8, CRLF2, and CD40L (Th2 inflammatory receptor). Targeting LNC_000127 may effectively reduce Th2 inflammation in eosinophilic asthma [52]. It has been demonstrated that induced pluripotent stem cells (iPSCs)-mesenchymal stem cells (MSCs) can effectively inhibit airway allergic inflammation in mice, and significantly reduce the expression levels of immunoglobulin (Ig) E and Th2 cytokines [53]. Further studies by Wang et al. [54] found that lncRNA MM9lincrnaexon12105 + and AK089315 were up-regulated in a model of ova-induced asthma. These two lncRNAs may be the main therapeutic targets of induced pluripotent stem cell mesenchymal stem cells (iPSC-MSCs) and may be involved in the regulation of Th2 type inflammation in asthma. This study provides an important basis for the study of the potential mechanisms of airway allergic inflammation and iPSC-MSC immune regulation, and these abnormal lncRNAs may become potential targets of allergic inflammation and iPSC-MSC mediated immune regulation. Wang et al. [55] conducted next-generation sequencing analysis of lncRNA and mRNAs on CD4 + T cells from ovalbumin-induced acute asthma mice and control mice, constructed co-expression networks of lncRNA and mRNAs, and found that lncRNA Fantom3_9230106C11 was decreased in Th2 cells. Further qRT-PCR verification showed that lncRNA Fantom3_9230106C11 could regulate the differentiation of Th2 cells. This study provides a platform to elucidate the role of lncRNA in Th2 differentiation and the pathogenesis of asthma. The role of Th2-mediated lncRNA in asthma are summarized in the **Table 2** (**Figure 2**).

Altered lncRNA	Expression pattern	Targets/ Regulators	Signaling Pathway	Function	Ref
MALTA1	Up-regulated		MALAT1 / miR-155 / CTLA-4	regulate Th1 / Th2 balance in asthma	[50]
lncRNA PVT1	Up-regulated	—	lncRNA PVT1-miR-15a-5p-PI3K/AKT/ mTOR axis	regulate Th1 / Th2 balance in asthma	[51]
LNC_000127	Up-regulated	—	—	reduce Th2 inflammation	[52]
MM9lincrnaexon12105 + and AK089315	Up-regulated	—	—	regulate Th2-type inflammation in asthma.	[54]
lncRNA Fantom3_9230106C11	Down-regulated	—		Regulate the differentiation of Th2 cells.	[55]

Table 2.
lncRNA regulate Th2 response in asthma.

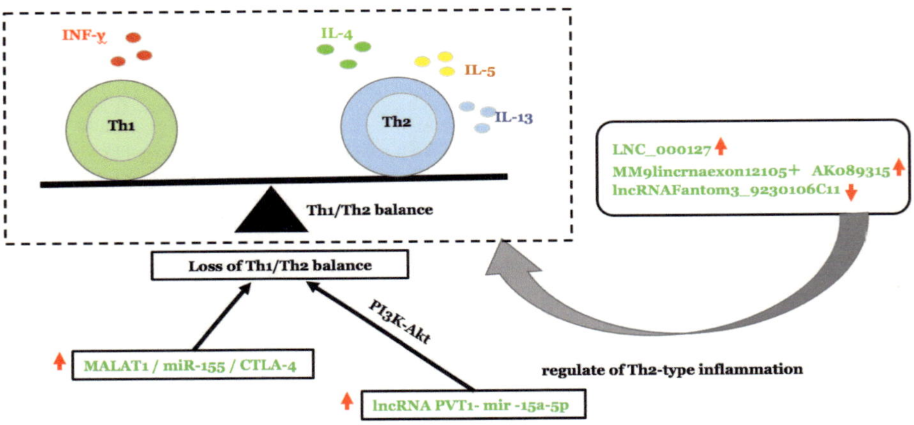

Figure 2.
lncRNA regulate Th2 response in asthma. MALAT1 sponging miR-155 could alter the Th1/Th2 balance within CD4+ T cells through CTLA-4 dependent mechanism. lncRNA PVT1-miR-15a-5p axis promoted Th1/Th2 imbalance in CD4 + T cells by activating the PI3K-Akt- signaling pathway. LNC_000127, MM9lincrnaexon12105 + and AK089315 and lncRNA Fantom3_9230106C11 primarily regulate the Th2-type inflammation.

4. circRNAs regulate Th2 response in asthma

CircRNAs compose a novel class of ncRNAs characterized by covalently closed-loop structures [56]. CircRNAs typically act as molecular sponges to bind and inhibit the transcription or activity of microRNAs (miRNAs), thereby affecting downstream mRNA expression [57]. CircRNAs are involved in the pathogenesis of various diseases [58]. The role of circRNA in asthma regulation is still in its infancy, and there are relatively few studies on the role of circRNA in the pathogenesis of asthma, especially Th2 inflammation in asthma.

Huang et al. [59] confirmed the expression of hsa_circ_0002594 in CD4 + T cells in asthmatic patients and healthy subjects by quantitative real-time PCR (qRT-PCR) using circRNA microarray analysis (such as a student's *t* test, nonparametric tests, Spearman's rank-order correlation, Fisher's exact test, and the generation of receiver operating characteristic curves). Their data suggest that hsa_circ_0002594 is upregulated in CD4 + T cells of asthmatic patients, which may have potential value in the diagnosis and treatment of Th2-mediated allergic asthma. In a mouse model of HDM-induced asthma, the results revealed that the relative expression levels of circ_0000629 and circ_0000455 in the asthma group were significantly increased compared with those animals in the control group, whereas the expression levels of circ_0000454 and circ_0000723 were significantly decreased [60]. The circRNA-miRNA regulatory network indicated that two of the downregulated circRNAs (circ_0001454 and circ_0000723) targeted miR-146b and miR-214, and two of these upregulated circRNAs (circ_0000455 and circ_0000629) could target miR-29b and miR-15a [60]. The expression levels of inducible co-stimulator, a target gene of miR-29b, were also previously shown to be elevated in the lungs of asthmatic mice, and promoted Th2 cytokine production and eosinophilic inflammation [61]. Furthermore, vascular endothelial growth factor, which is a target gene of mir-15a, was shown to be overexpressed in cases of Th2-mediated lung inflammation, such as asthma, and induced an asthma-like phenotype [62]. By contrast, two of the downregulated circRNAs (circ_0001454 and circ_0000723) targeted miR-146b and miR-214, respectively, which were previously shown to be positively associated with asthma [34, 63]. Huang et al. found that hsa_circ_0005519 may induce IL-13 and IL-6 expression by regulating hsa-let-7a-5p in $CD4^+$ T cells to affect asthma. And hsa_circ_0005519 may be a potential biomarker of asthma [64]. The role of Th2-mediated circRNAs in asthma are summarized in the **Table 3** (**Figure 3**).

Altered circRNA	Expressi-on pattern	Targets/ Regul-ators	Signaling Pathway	Function	Ref
hsa_circ_0002594	Up-regulated	—	—	diagnosis and treatment of Th2-mediated allergic asthma	[59]
circ_0000629	Up-regulated	miR-29b, miR-15a	—	Regulate Th2 cytokine production	[34, 60–63]
circ_0000455	Up-regulated				
circ_0001454	Down-regulated	miR-146b, miR-214	—		
circ_0000723	Down-regulated				
hsa_circ_0005519	Up-regulated	Hsa-let-7a-5p	—	relieve suppression for IL-13/IL-6 in $CD4^+$ T cells.	[64]

Table 3.
circRNAs regulate Th2 response in asthma.

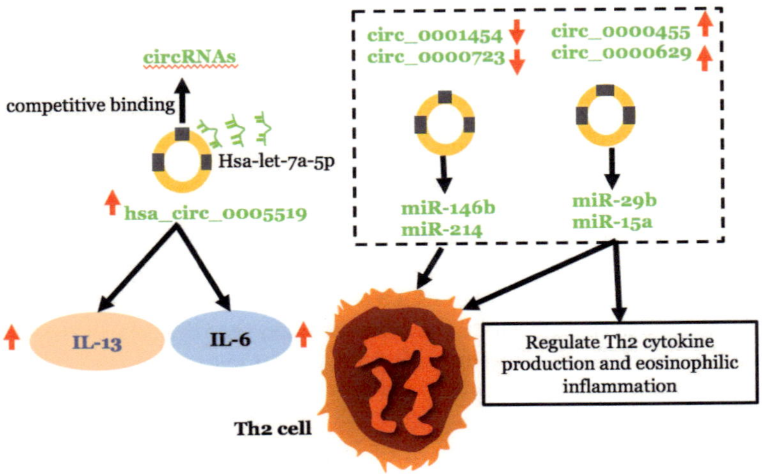

Figure 3.
circRNAs regulate Th2 response in asthma. Hsa_circ_0005519 functions as an endogenous hsa-let-7a-5p sponge to regulate the hsa-let-7a-5p/IL-13/IL-6 pathway in CD4$^+$ T cells. Two down-regulated circRNAs (circ_0001454 and circ_0000723) targeted miR-146b and miR-214, while two up-regulated circRNAs (circ_0000455 and circ_0000629) targeted miR-29b and miR-15a. These four circRNAs regulate TH2 cytokine production by targeting miRNA.

5. Summary

NcRNAs display a wide range of functions, and each ncRNA has its own characteristics. This chapter mainly summarized the regulation of Th2 differentiation and immune response in asthma and experimental models of disease.

The role of miRNA in regulating Th2 cell-mediated inflammation in asthma is mainly reflected in several aspects: regulating Th1/Th2 balance, influencing cytokine secretion and regulating the activation state of T cells. The pathway of regulation can be that a single miRNA regulates one or more mRNAs, or multiple miRNAs of one or more gene clusters synergistically act on one or more mRNAs to exert biological effects. LncRNA plays a similar role to miRNA in regulating Th2 cell-mediated inflammation in asthma, affecting its activation, transformation and cytokine secretion. Most of the existing studies only analyzed the expression profile of lncRNA and identified the differentially expressed lncRNA molecules, but did not conduct in-depth study on its precise molecular mechanism. CircRNAs may play important roles in Th2 cells differentiation and, thus, play regulatory roles in Th2 cell-mediated inflammation in asthma. They can act as competitive endogenous RNAs (ceRNAs, which can regulate each other by competitively binding common microRNA response elements) of miRNAs to exert their biological effects, but the specific mechanism needs to be further studied.

In conclusion, miRNA, lncRNA and circRNA play important roles in regulation of Th2 cell function in asthma. However, the exact molecular mechanism of ncRNA in the regulation of TH2 cell function in asthma remains to be determined. Therefore, how to find out functional ncRNAs and elucidate their precise functions present the difficulties and challenges in the study of ncRNAs in this field. In future, more and more ncRNAs involved in the pathogenesis of asthma will be discovered, and the role of ncRNAs in the inflammatory process mediated by Th2 cells will be revealed. This will provide new details in the pathogenesis of asthma, and will help to develop new biomarkers and molecular targets for the diagnosis, classification, and treatment of asthma.

Conflict of interest

The authors declare no conflict of interest.

Author details

Yanhua Niu[1], Chao Wang[1], Xiaoyan Dong[1*] and Nanbert Zhong[2*]

1 Department of Pulmonary, Shanghai Children's Hospital, Shanghai Jiaotong University, Shanghai, China

2 New York State Institute for Basic Research in Developmental Disabilities, Staten Island, NY, USA

*Address all correspondence to: dong_x_y0305@126.com
and dongxy@shchildren.com.cn

References

[1] Pavord ID, Beasley R, Agusti A, Anderson GP, Bel E, Brusselle G, Cullinan P, Custovic A, Ducharme FM, Fahy JV, Frey U, Gibson P, Heaney LG, Holt PG, Humbert M, Lloyd CM, Marks G, Martinez FD, Sly PD, von Mutius E, Wenzel S, Zar HJ, Bush A. After asthma: redefining airways diseases. Lancet. 2018 Jan 27;391(10118):350-400.

[2] E.D. Bateman, S.S. Hurd, P.J. Barnes, J. Bousquet, J.M. Drazen, J.M. FitzGerald, P. Gibson, K. Ohta, P. O'Byrne, S.E. Pedersen, E. Pizzichini, S.D. Sullivan, S.E. Wenzel, H.J. Zar, Global strategy for asthma management and prevention: GINA executive summary, Eur Respir J, 31 (2008) 143-178.

[3] Ghafouri-Fard S, Shoorei H, Taheri M, Sanak M. Emerging role of non-coding RNAs in allergic disorders. Biomed Pharmacother. 2020 Oct; 130:110615.

[4] Moharamoghli M, Hassan-Zadeh V, Dolatshahi E, Alizadeh Z, Farazmand A. The expression of GAS5, THRIL, and RMRP lncRNAs is increased in T cells of patients with rheumatoid arthritis. Clin Rheumatol. 2019 Nov;38(11):3073-3080.

[5] Zhou R, Wu Y, Wang W, Su W, Liu Y, Wang Y, Fan C, Li X, Li G, Li Y, Xiong W, Zeng Z. Circular RNAs (circRNAs) in cancer. Cancer Lett. 2018 Jul 1; 425:134-142.

[6] Foster PS, Maltby S, Rosenberg HF, Tay HL, Hogan SP, Collison AM, Yang M, Kaiko GE, Hansbro PM, Kumar RK, Mattes J. Modeling T_H 2 responses and airway inflammation to understand fundamental mechanisms regulating the pathogenesis of asthma. Immunol Rev. 2017 Jul;278(1):20-40.

[7] Mukherjee M, Nair P. Autoimmune Responses in Severe Asthma. Allergy Asthma Immunol Res. 2018 Sep;10(5):428-447.

[8] Dong C, Flavell RA. Th1 and Th2 cells. Curr Opin Hematol. 2001 Jan;8(1):47-51.

[9] Kannan AK, Sahu N, Mohanan S, Mohinta S, August A. IL-2-inducible T-cell kinase modulates TH2-mediated allergic airway inflammation by suppressing IFN-γ in naive CD4+ T cells. J Allergy Clin Immunol. 2013 Oct;132(4):811-20. e1-5.

[10] Zhang B, Farwell MA. microRNAs: a new emerging class of players for disease diagnostics and gene therapy. J Cell Mol Med. 2008 Jan-Feb;12(1):3-21.

[11] Pauley KM, Cha S, Chan EK. MicroRNA in autoimmunity and autoimmune diseases. J Autoimmun. 2009 May-Jun;32(3-4):189-94.

[12] Gebert LFR, MacRae IJ. Regulation of microRNA function in animals. Nat Rev Mol Cell Biol. 2019 Jan;20(1):21-37.

[13] Rebane A, Akdis CA. MicroRNAs in allergy and asthma. Curr Allergy Asthma Rep. 2014 Apr;14(4):424.

[14] Collison A, Mattes J, Plank M, Foster PS. Inhibition of house dust mite-induced allergic airways disease by antagonism of microRNA-145 is comparable to glucocorticoid treatment. J Allergy Clin Immunol. 2011 Jul;128(1):160-167.e4.

[15] Pua HH, Steiner DF, Patel S, Gonzalez JR, Ortiz-Carpena JF, Kageyama R, Chiou NT, Gallman A, de Kouchkovsky D, Jeker LT, McManus MT, Erle DJ, Ansel KM. MicroRNAs 24 and 27 Suppress Allergic Inflammation and Target a Network of Regulators of T Helper 2 Cell-Associated Cytokine Production. Immunity. 2016 Apr 19;44(4):821-32.

[16] Lu TX, Munitz A, Rothenberg ME. MicroRNA-21 is up-regulated in allergic airway inflammation and regulates IL-12p35 expression. J Immunol. 2009 Apr 15;182(8):4994-5002.

[17] Panganiban RP, Pinkerton MH, Maru SY, Jefferson SJ, Roff AN, Ishmael FT. Differential microRNA epression in asthma and the role of miR-1248 in regulation of IL-5. Am J Clin Exp Immunol. 2012 Nov 15;1(2):154-65.

[18] Borish L, Aarons A, Rumbyrt J, Cvietusa P, Negri J, Wenzel S. Interleukin-10 regulation in normal subjects and patients with asthma. J Allergy Clin Immunol. 1996 Jun;97(6):1288-96.

[19] Sharma A, Kumar M, Ahmad T, Mabalirajan U, Aich J, Agrawal A, Ghosh B. Antagonism of mmu-mir-106a attenuates asthma features in allergic murine model. J Appl Physiol (1985). 2012 Aug;113(3):459-64.

[20] Simpson LJ, Patel S, Bhakta NR, Choy DF, Brightbill HD, Ren X, Wang Y, Pua HH, Baumjohann D, Montoya MM, Panduro M, Remedios KA, Huang X, Fahy JV, Arron JR, Woodruff PG, Ansel KM. A microRNA upregulated in asthma airway T cells promotes TH2 cytokine production. Nat Immunol. 2014 Dec;15(12):1162-70.

[21] Han S, Ma C, Bao L, Lv L, Huang M. miR-146a Mimics Attenuate Allergic Airway Inflammation by Impacted Group 2 Innate Lymphoid Cells in an Ovalbumin-Induced Asthma Mouse Model. Int Arch Allergy Immunol. 2018;177(4):302-310.

[22] Zech A, Ayata CK, Pankratz F, Meyer A, Baudiß K, Cicko S, Yegutkin GG, Grundmann S, Idzko M. MicroRNA-155 modulates P2R signaling and Th2 priming of dendritic cells during allergic airway inflammation in mice. Allergy. 2015 Sep;70(9):1121-9.

[23] Zhou H, Li J, Gao P, Wang Q, Zhang J. miR-155: A Novel Target in Allergic Asthma. Int J Mol Sci. 2016 Oct 24;17(10):1773.

[24] Kumar M, Ahmad T, Sharma A, Mabalirajan U, Kulshreshtha A, Agrawal A, Ghosh B. Let-7 microRNA-mediated regulation of IL-13 and allergic airway inflammation. J Allergy Clin Immunol. 2011 Nov;128(5):1077-85. e 1-10.

[25] Jin R, Hu S, Liu X, Guan R, Lu L, Lin R. Intranasal instillation of miR-410 targeting IL-4/IL-13 attenuates airway inflammation in OVA-induced asthmatic mice. Mol Med Rep. 2019 Feb;19(2):895-900.

[26] Huang XP, Qin CY, Gao YM. miR-135a inhibits airway inflammatory response in asthmatic mice via regulating JAK/STAT signaling pathway. Braz J Med Biol Res. 2021 Jan 15;54(3): e10023.

[27] Grünig G, Warnock M, Wakil AE, Venkayya R, Brombacher F, Rennick DM, Sheppard D, Mohrs M, Donaldson DD, Locksley RM, Corry DB. Requirement for IL-13 independently of IL-4 in experimental asthma. Science. 1998 Dec 18;282(5397):2261-3.

[28] Wills-Karp M, Luyimbazi J, Xu X, Schofield B, Neben TY, Karp CL, Donaldson DD. Interleukin-13: central mediator of allergic asthma. Science. 1998 Dec 18;282(5397):2258-61.

[29] Kuperman DA, Huang X, Koth LL, Chang GH, Dolganov GM, Zhu Z, Elias JA, Sheppard D, Erle DJ. Direct effects of interleukin-13 on epithelial cells cause airway hyperreactivity and mucus overproduction in asthma. Nat Med. 2002 Aug;8(8):885-9.

[30] Solberg OD, Ostrin EJ, Love MI, Peng JC, Bhakta NR, Hou L, Nguyen C, Solon M, Nguyen C, Barczak AJ,

Zlock LT, Blagev DP, Finkbeiner WE, Ansel KM, Arron JR, Erle DJ, Woodruff PG. Airway epithelial miRNA expression is altered in asthma. Am J Respir Crit Care Med. 2012 Nov 15;186(10):965-74.

[31] Zhang K, Liang Y, Feng Y, Wu W, Zhang H, He J, Hu Q, Zhao J, Xu Y, Liu Z, Zhen G. Decreased epithelial and sputum miR-221-3p associates with airway eosinophilic inflammation and CXCL17 expression in asthma. Am J Physiol Lung Cell Mol Physiol. 2018 Aug 1;315(2): L253-L264.

[32] Shi ZG, Sun Y, Wang KS, Jia JD, Yang J, Li YN. Effects of miR-26a/miR-146a/miR-31 on airway inflammation of asthma mice and asthma children. Eur Rev Med Pharmacol Sci. 2019 Jun;23(12):5432-5440.

[33] Kılıç A, Santolini M, Nakano T, Schiller M, Teranishi M, Gellert P, Ponomareva Y, Braun T, Uchida S, Weiss ST, Sharma A, Renz H. A systems immunology approach identifies the collective impact of 5 miRs in Th2 inflammation. JCI Insight. 2018 Jun 7;3(11): e97503.

[34] Qiu YY, Zhang YW, Qian XF, Bian T. miR-371, miR-138, miR-544, miR-145, and miR-214 could modulate Th1/Th2 balance in asthma through the combinatorial regulation of Runx3. Am J Transl Res. 2017 Jul 15;9(7): 3184-3199.

[35] Steiner DF, Thomas MF, Hu JK, Yang Z, Babiarz JE, Allen CD, Matloubian M, Blelloch R, Ansel KM. MicroRNA-29 regulates T-box transcription factors and interferon-γ production in helper T cells. Immunity. 2011 Aug 26;35(2):169-81.

[36] Yan J, Zhang X, Sun S, Yang T, Yang J, Wu G, Qiu Y, Yin Y, Xu W. miR-29b Reverses T helper 1 cells/T helper 2 cells Imbalance and Alleviates Airway Eosinophils Recruitment in OVA-Induced Murine Asthma by Targeting Inducible Co-Stimulator. Int Arch Allergy Immunol. 2019;180(3):182-194.

[37] Bartel S, La Grutta S, Cilluffo G, Perconti G, Bongiovanni A, Giallongo A, Behrends J, Kruppa J, Hermann S, Chiang D, Pfaffl MW, Krauss-Etschmann S. Human airway epithelial extracellular vesicle miRNA signature is altered upon asthma development. Allergy. 2020 Feb;75(2):346-356.

[38] Collison A, Herbert C, Siegle JS, Mattes J, Foster PS, Kumar RK. Altered expression of microRNA in the airway wall in chronic asthma: miR-126 as a potential therapeutic target. BMC Pulm Med. 2011 May 23; 11:29.

[39] Mattes J, Collison A, Plank M, Phipps S, Foster PS. Antagonism of microRNA-126 suppresses the effector function of TH2 cells and the development of allergic airways disease. Proc Natl Acad Sci U S A. 2009 Nov 3;106(44):18704-9.

[40] Wang T, Zhou Q, Shang Y. Downregulation of miRNA-451a Promotes the Differentiation of CD4+ T Cells towards Th2 Cells by Upregulating ETS1 in Childhood Asthma. J Innate Immun. 2021;13(1):38-48.

[41] Wang Z, Ji N, Chen Z, Sun Z, Wu C, Yu W, Hu F, Huang M, Zhang M. MiR-1165-3p Suppresses Th2 Differentiation via Targeting IL-13 and PPM1A in a Mouse Model of Allergic Airway Inflammation. Allergy Asthma Immunol Res. 2020 Sep;12(5):859-876.

[42] Zhang X, Zhao X, Sun H, Yan Y, Huang L, Gu W, Jiang W, Wang Y, Zhu C, Ji W, Hao C, Chen Z. The role of miR-29c/B7-H3 axis in children with allergic asthma. J Transl Med. 2018 Aug 3;16(1):218.

[43] Sawant DV, Wu H, Kaplan MH, Dent AL. The Bcl6 target gene microRNA-21 promotes Th2 differentiation by a T cell intrinsic pathway. Mol Immunol. 2013 Jul;54(3-4):435-42.

[44] Long CM, Lukomska E, Marshall NB, Nayak A, Anderson SE. Potential Inhibitory Influence of miRNA 210 on Regulatory T Cells during Epicutaneous Chemical Sensitization. Genes (Basel). 2016 Dec 27;8(1):9.

[45] Yang L, Lin C, Jin C, Yang JC, Tanasa B, Li W, Merkurjev D, Ohgi KA, Meng D, Zhang J, Evans CP, Rosenfeld MG. lncRNA-dependent mechanisms of androgen-receptor-regulated gene activation programs. Nature. 2013 Aug 29;500(7464):598-602.

[46] Kim J, Kim KM, Noh JH, Yoon JH, Abdelmohsen K, Gorospe M. Long noncoding RNAs in diseases of aging. Biochim Biophys Acta. 2016 Jan;1859(1):209-21.

[47] Hu G, Tang Q, Sharma S, Yu F, Escobar TM, Muljo SA, Zhu J, Zhao K. Expression and regulation of intergenic long noncoding RNAs during T cell development and differentiation. Nat Immunol. 2013 Nov;14(11):1190-8.

[48] Narożna B, Langwiński W, Szczepankiewicz A. Non-Coding RNAs in Pediatric Airway Diseases. Genes (Basel). 2017 Nov 27;8(12):348.

[49] Ji P, Diederichs S, Wang W, Böing S, Metzger R, Schneider PM, Tidow N, Brandt B, Buerger H, Bulk E, Thomas M, Berdel WE, Serve H, Müller-Tidow C. MALAT-1, a novel noncoding RNA, and thymosin beta4 predict metastasis and survival in early-stage non-small cell lung cancer. Oncogene. 2003 Sep 11;22(39):8031-41.

[50] Liang Z, Tang F. The potency of lncRNA MALAT1/miR-155/CTLA4 axis in altering Th1/Th2 balance of asthma. Biosci Rep. 2020 Feb 28;40(2): BSR20190397.

[51] Wei Y, Han B, Dai W, Guo S, Zhang C, Zhao L, Gao Y, Jiang Y, Kong X. Exposure to ozone impacted Th1/Th2 imbalance of CD^{4+} T cells and apoptosis of ASMCs underlying asthmatic progression by activating lncRNA PVT1-miR-15a-5p/miR-29c-3p signaling. Aging (Albany NY). 2020 Nov 20;12(24):25229-25255.

[52] Zhu Y, Mao D, Gao W, Han G, Hu H. Analysis of lncRNA Expression in Patients With Eosinophilic and Neutrophilic Asthma Focusing on LNC_000127. Front Genet. 2019 Mar 19;10: 141.

[53] Y.Q. Sun, M.X. Deng, J. He, Q.X. Zeng, W. Wen, D.S. Wong, H.F. Tse, G. Xu, Q. Lian, J. Shi, Q.L. Fu, Human pluripotent stem cell-derived mesenchymal stem cells prevent allergic airway inflammation in mice, Stem Cells, 30 (2012) 2692-2699.

[54] Wang SY, Fan XL, Yu QN, Deng MX, Sun YQ, Gao WX, Li CL, Shi JB, Fu QL. The lncRNAs involved in mouse airway allergic inflammation following induced pluripotent stem cell-mesenchymal stem cell treatment. Stem Cell Res Ther. 2017 Jan 6;8(1):2.

[55] Wang Z, Ji N, Chen Z, Wu C, Sun Z, Yu W, Hu F, Huang M, Zhang M. Next Generation Sequencing for Long Non-coding RNAs Profile for $CD4^+$ T Cells in the Mouse Model of Acute Asthma. Front Genet. 2019 Jun 7; 10:545.

[56] Memczak S, Jens M, Elefsinioti A, Torti F, Krueger J, Rybak A, Maier L, Mackowiak SD, Gregersen LH, Munschauer M, Loewer A, Ziebold U, Landthaler M, Kocks C, le Noble F, Rajewsky N. Circular RNAs are a large class of animal RNAs with regulatory potency. Nature. 2013 Mar 21;495(7441):333-8.

[57] Hansen TB, Jensen TI, Clausen BH, Bramsen JB, Finsen B, Damgaard CK, Kjems J. Natural RNA circles function as efficient microRNA sponges. Nature. 2013 Mar 21;495(7441):384-8.

[58] Vidal AF, Sandoval GT, Magalhães L, Santos SE, Ribeiro-dos-Santos Â. Circular RNAs as a new field in gene regulation and their implications in translational research. Epigenomics. 2016 Apr;8(4):551-62.

[59] Huang Z, Fu B, Qi X, Xu Y, Mou Y, Zhou M, Cao Y, Wu G, Xie J, Zhao J, Wang Y, Xiong W. Diagnostic and Therapeutic Value of Hsa_circ_0002594 for T Helper 2-Mediated Allergic Asthma. Int Arch Allergy Immunol. 2020 Dec 16:1-11.

[60] Bao H, Zhou Q, Li Q, Niu M, Chen S, Yang P, Liu Z, Xia L. Differentially expressed circular RNAs in a murine asthma model. Mol Med Rep. 2020 Dec;22(6):5412-5422.

[61] Gonzalo JA, Tian J, Delaney T, Corcoran J, Rottman JB, Lora J, Al-garawi A, Kroczek R, Gutierrez-Ramos JC, Coyle AJ. ICOS is critical for T helper cell-mediated lung mucosal inflammatory responses. Nat Immunol. 2001 Jul;2(7):597-604.

[62] Lee CG, Link H, Baluk P, Homer RJ, Chapoval S, Bhandari V, Kang MJ, Cohn L, Kim YK, McDonald DM, Elias JA. Vascular endothelial growth factor (VEGF) induces remodeling and enhances TH2-mediated sensitization and inflammation in the lung. Nat Med. 2004 Oct;10(10):1095-103.

[63] Feng MJ, Shi F, Qiu C, Peng WK. MicroRNA-181a, –146a and -146b in spleen CD4+ T lymphocytes play proinflammatory roles in a murine model of asthma. Int Immunopharmacol. 2012 Jul;13(3):347-53.

[64] Huang Z, Cao Y, Zhou M, Qi X, Fu B, Mou Y, Wu G, Xie J, Zhao J, Xiong W. Hsa_circ_0005519 increases IL-13/IL-6 by regulating hsa-let-7a-5p in $CD4^+$ T cells to affect asthma. Clin Exp Allergy. 2019 Aug;49(8):1116-1127.

Chapter 5

Asthma Phenotypes and Current Biological Treatments

Aşkın Gülşen

Abstract

Asthma is a heterogeneous disease characterized by bronchial hyperreactivity, chronic airway inflammation, and reversible airflow obstruction, and it affects individuals in all age groups. In recent years, the concept of intrinsic and extrinsic asthma as per the former classification has been replaced by endotypic and phenotypic definitions. However, the two main asthma endotypes described and have simplified its classification. These endotypes, "Th2-high" and "Th2-low", are based on various measurements obtained for different biological materials, including blood, bronchial and sputum samples. The definitions of asthma is useful for targeted and individualized treatments, estimating the treatment response and prognosis. In the field of respiratory medicine, biological drugs (BDs) have shown rapid evolution and positive developments in the last 10 years, particularly for the treatment of asthma, interstitial lung disease, and lung cancer. However, because of the increasing number of BDs and associated studies, it has become very difficult to update treatment guidelines on a regular basis. BDs are used for patients with difficult-to-treat, moderate to severe, and/or uncontrolled allergic asthma. Here we present a review of current asthma phenotypes and the role, efficacy, and side effects of BDs used for the treatment of these conditions.

Keywords: Asthma, phenotype, endotype, biological treatment, biologics

1. Introduction

Asthma is a heterogeneous disease characterized by bronchial hyperreactivity, chronic airway inflammation, and reversible airflow obstruction, and it affects individuals in all age groups [1]. In recent years, studies on endotype and phenotype have intensified, and many different types have been identified. Symptom control is generally achieved with the use of inhaled corticosteroids (ICSs), although biological drugs (BDs) are used for patients with difficult-to-treat, moderate to severe, and/or uncontrolled allergic asthma [1], as these patient groups largely benefit from BD therapies. BDs, also known as biologics, encompass a number of agents that are rapidly growing and expanding their range of use. These drugs generally act on cell surface receptors or by interacting with a specific cytokine and are produced either directly from living sources (animal, human or microorganism) or by synthesizing from different cell cultures [2]. Currently, they are widely used in the fields of oncology, rheumatology, dermatology, and organ transplantation, and their indications include organ-specific cancers, psoriasis, rheumatoid arthritis, psoriatic arthritis, inflammatory bowel disease, chronic urticaria, multiple sclerosis, and transplants [3]. In the field of respiratory medicine, biologics have shown rapid evolution and positive developments in the last 10 years, particularly for the treatment of severe uncontrolled asthma, interstitial lung disease, and lung cancer. In this review, we will evaluate the current updates of asthma phenotypes and the role, efficacy, and side effects of BDs used for the treatment of these conditions.

2. Endotypes and phenotypes of asthma

The concept of intrinsic and extrinsic asthma as per the former classification has been replaced by endotypic and phenotypic definitions. However, a lack of clear classification system leads to a confusion and limitation in treatment. The current Global Initiative for Asthma (GINA) 2020 guideline mentions phenotypic differences in allergic asthma, nonallergic asthma, late-onset asthma, asthma with fixed airflow limitation, and asthma with obesity [1]. Although this guideline does not provide much details on asthma phenotyping, it mentions that further studies are necessary. Following the introduction of the phenotype concept, in 2006 Simpson et al. [4] conducted a study to fully characterize asthma based on the airway inflammatory type. The authors performed induced sputum analysis and divided the patients into the following four subgroups according to the dominant inflammatory cell type: a. neutrophilic, where neutrophils are >61% and the total cell count is >10 million cells/g; b. eosinophilic, where eosinophils are >1.9–3%; c. mixed granulocytic, where there is an increase in both neutrophils and eosinophils; and d. paucigranulocytic, where both neutrophils and eosinophils are within the normal range [4]. It is known that this classification of airway inflammation in asthma is important in predicting the clinical significance and response to BDs. Moreover, the authors reported that the rate of eosinophils in induced sputum is homogeneous and reproducible for eosinophilic asthma and heterogeneous for the other non-eosinophilic types of disease, and that further classification can be based on the presence of neutrophils [4].

However, a study involving 726 patients from the Severe Asthma Research Program (SARP) cohort was performed, and five main groups were identified [5] as follows: group 1, early-onset atopic asthma, control with two or fewer controlling drugs, normal lung function; group 2, early-onset atopic asthma, preserved lung function [65%; forced expiratory volume in 1 s (FEV1), >80% predicted], control with three or more controlling drugs (29% patients); group 3, late-onset nonatopic asthma, moderate decrease in FEV1, frequent oral corticosteroid (OCS) and ICS use for the treatment of exacerbations; group 4, early-onset atopic asthma with severely compromised pulmonary function (57% of the mean FEV1); and group 5, late-onset asthma, most severe airflow limitation (43% of the mean FEV1), less atopic patients with varying degrees of susceptibility to bronchodilator therapy. Then, subgroup analysis was performed as an extension of the same study, and the importance of eosinophil (≥2%) and neutrophil (≥40%) percentages in the sputum was emphasized [6]. From these findings, it was understood that asthma is a very heterogeneous disease with inflammatory and noninflammatory mechanisms. Considering the role of Type 2 T-helper cell (Th2) lymphocytes in eosinophilic airway inflammation, clinical studies have been inclined toward this topic. However, the two main asthma endotypes described in recent years have simplified its classification [7–9]. These endotypes, "Th2-high" and "Th2-low", are based on various measurements obtained for different biological materials, including blood, and bronchial, and sputum samples [10]. The Th2-high type is generally characterized by increased eosinophils in the patient's sputum and respiratory tract, while the Th2-low type is characterized by increased neutrophils or by the presence of a paucigranulocytic pattern [10]. The Th2-high patient group can be identified by some biomarkers, particularly an elevated blood eosinophil count of >300 cells/mL, and these patients have shown a good response to treatment with BDs [10]. There are no defined biomarkers for the Th2-low endotype, so this phenotype is often identified by the absence of Th2-high biomarkers. Moreover, these patients do not respond well to steroids [10].

Currently, the serum immunglobulin (Ig)-E concentration and the number of peripheral blood eosinophilis are generally used to determine the response of patients with BD treatment [7, 9]. A combination of Th2 biomarkers such as interleukin (IL)-4, IL-5, and IL-13 is also considered to be a credible predictor of peripheral blood eosinophilia and eosinophilic inflammation [11]. Several other biomarkers that can be used include the following: **a.)** periostin, which plays a role in late-onset asthma and determines eosinophilic inflammation; **b.)** eotaxin-2, which determines eosinophilic inflammation; **c.)** L-arginine and leptin, which are associated with obesity-related asthma; **d.)** Chlamydia pneumonia antibodies (IgG, IgA, and IgE), which are associated with severe and obstructive asthma; **e.)** *Staphylococcus aureus* enterotoxin-IgE, which is associated with severe asthma, hospitalizations, OCS use, and lower FEV1; and f.) thymic stromal lymphopoietin (TSLP), which may play a role in sputum eosinophil elevation in smokers with asthma, thus helping in identification of this patient group [12]. Other investigations that help to improve endotyping include the measurements of the fraction of exhaled nitric oxide (FeNO) and skin prick tests [7]. The levels of allergen-specific antibodies may be considered clinically important in patients with asthma and atopy even if they are not used for endotyping. The World Asthma Phenotypes (WASP) study was initiated in 2016 and conducted in five countries; the results are awaited [13]. The aim of this study was to evaluate and compare detailed biomarker and clinical information, the distribution of disease phenotypes, and the risk factors and characteristics for each phenotype, including clinical severity.

In summary, the definition of asthma phenotypes and endotypes is useful for estimating the treatment response and prognosis. This approach has resulted in targeted and individualized treatments for patients (**Figure 1**).

2.1 Th2-high endotype

The asthma phenotypes that can be included in this group include aspirin-associated asthma, allergic bronchopulmonary mycosis (ABPM), early-onset (preschool wheezer) asthma, adult-onset asthma, late-onset severe hypereosinophilic asthma, and IgE-mediated occupational asthma (**Table 1**). These phenotypes can be classified under the Th2-high endotype because of the presence of significant allergic symptoms and eosinophilic inflammation.

Patients with aspirin-related or aspirin-sensitive asthma often present at polyclinics with nasal polyposis and severe rhinosinusitis [7]. The most important biomarkers are urinary leukotriene and blood eosinophils, although periostin may also be elevated [14]. The ABPM phenotype includes patients with adult-onset, severe asthma attacks and increased mucus production [7], and blood eosinophil counts, high IgE levels, high FeNO values, allergen-specific IgE, and skin prick tests can be used for identification [14]. Preschool wheezers are children with a family history of asthma who experience more than three episodes per year and often exhibit blood eosinophilia (>4%) and aeroallergen-specific IgE positivity [14]. The adult-onset allergic asthma phenotype includes patients having asthma since childhood, with symptoms of allergen-related rhinitis, positive skin prick tests, high IgE levels, and high FeNO values [7, 14]. The severe late-onset hypereosinophilic asthma phenotype includes nonatopic patients with severe exacerbations and peripheral blood eosinophilia [7, 14]. Patients with IgE-mediated occupational asthma, wherein asthma symptoms develop after the start of a new occupation or job, may also be included in

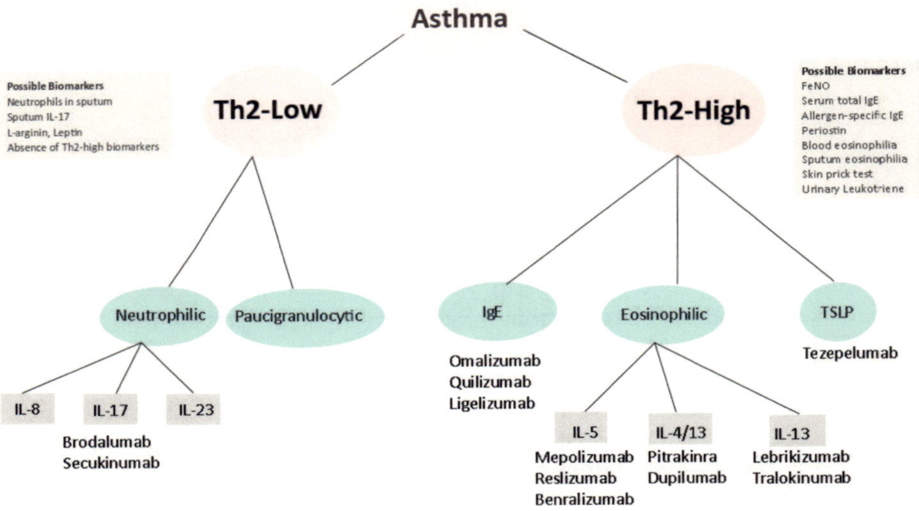

Figure 1.
Asthma phenotypes and current targets for biological treatment. Th2, T-helper type 2 cell; IL, interleukin; IgE, immunoglobulin E; TSLP, tymic stromal lymphopoietin; ACO, Asthma COPD overlap.

Phenotype	Clinical presentation	Biomarkers
Aspirin-Associated [7, 14]	Nasal polyposis, rhinosinusitis, adult onset,. **Therapy:** 5-LO or LTRA inhibitors	Urinary Leukotriene, increased periostin levels
Allergic Bronchopulmonary Mycosis [7, 14]	Mucus production, severe, adult onset, less reversibility, poor prognosis, **Therapy:** GKs, antifungals and biologics	High FeNO, High serum total IgE, High Aspergillus IgE, Positive Aspergillus skin testing.
Early Onset (preschool Wheezer) [14]	>3 episodes per year, early onset, history of asthma in parents **Therapy:** Daily inhaled GKs, LTRA, biologics	High FeNO, periostin, High IgE and Aeroallergen-specific IgE Eosinophils (often >4%) Positive Skin Pricktest,
Adult Onset [8]	Allergen associated symptoms/allergic rhinitis **Therapy:** GKs and biologics	High FeNO and total IgE, Positive Skin Pricktest,
Late Onset, severe and hypereosinophilic [7, 14]	Severe Exacerbations, non-atopic, GK-sensitive and often oral Gkk-dependent. **Therapy:** GKs and Anti-IL-5	High FeNO and eotaxins High Blood and Sputum Eosinophils,
Occupational, (IgE mediated) [15]	Asthmatic symptoms after onset new work **Therapy:** removal from exposure to the sensitizing agent	High FeNO, High IgE and allergen-specific IgE, sputum eosinophilia, Specific inhalation challenge, Peak expiratory flow

5-LO, 5-lipoxygenase; LT, leukotriene recepter antagonist; GK, Glucocorticoid; IgE,Immunglobulin E; FeNO, Fraction of exhaled nitric oxide in ppb; IL, Interleukin.

Table 1.
Possible Th2-high Endotypes of asthma.

this group. Specific inhalation challenge and peak expiratory flow measurement are required to diagnose these patients, along with high IgE levels, high allergen-specific IgE levels, high FeNO values, and sputum eosinophilia [15].

2.2 Th2-low endotype

This group includes asthma-COPD overlap (ACO; fixed obstruction) syndrome, late-onset nonatopic asthma, steroid-resistant or neutrophilic asthma, obesity related asthma, perimenstrual asthma, and non-IgE-mediated occupational asthma. Phenotypes induced by external factors, including exercise-induced asthma, cold-induced or cross-country skiers asthma, stress-induced asthma, and psychological asthma, may also be included in this group (**Table 2**). However, this classification needs to be improved by further research.

According to the current GINA guideline, the term ACOS is used for patients with chronic respiratory symptoms, exposure to a risk factor such as smoking, and a postbronchodilatator FEV1/forced vital capacity (FVC) of <0.7 [1]. Although the latter is not a well-known biomarker, the condition can be easily identified by using a questionnaire [1]. Late-onset nonatopic asthma generally affects women and adults.

Phenotype	Clinical presentation	Biomarkers
ACO or Fixed Obstruktion [1]	Chronic respiratory symptoms, exposure to a risk factor such as smoking, and post-bronchodilatator FEV1/FVC <0.7 Therapy: LABA + LAMA	—
Late Onset non-atopic [12, 16]	Particularly women, some adults, **Therapy:** require higher dose of ICS, relatively refractory to GKs	Absence of increase in sputum eosinophil count or FeNO
Poorly steroid responsive (neutrophilic) [7, 8]	Adult onset, low FEV1 and more Airtrapping, severe. **Therapy:** Macrolide, IL-17 antagonist	>76% neutrophils in sputum, IL-17
Obesity Related [12]	Often seen in obese women, less atopic, **Therapy:** Weight control	L-Arginin, Leptin
Pre- or perimenstrual [1]	A longer duration of Asthma, worsen in premenstrual phase, often dysmenorrhoe	—
Occupational (non-IgE mediated) [16]	Irritant-induced symptoms, poor prognosis, develops after acute high exposure to vapor, gas, fume, or smoke	Specific inhalation challenge. Peak expiratory flow
Asthma triggered by external factors		
Cold-Induced or Cross-Country Skiers [14]	Common upper respiratory tract infection, related to exercise and cold, poorly GKK respond **Therapy:** reducing cold exposure and training intensity	Normal FeNO, Normal blood eosinophil count, increased LT-E4 in urine
Exercise-Induced [17]	Develops due to increased catecholamines during exercise, resulting in increased airway resistance	—
Stress-Induced or Psychological [18]	After psychological stress, develop with the release of stress hormones	—

*ACO, Asthma-COPD-Overlap; LABA, long-acting beta agonist; LAMA, long-acting muscarinic antagonist; ICS, inhaled corticosteroids; FEV_1, forced expiratory volume in 1 s; FVC, orced vital capacity; See **Table 1** legend for expansion of other abbreviation.*

Table 2.
Possible Th2-low Endotypes of asthma.

Patients do not respond well to glucocorticoids and require high-dose ICSs [12]. This phenotype is similar to the obesity-associated phenotype. Although there is no biomarker, the absence of an increase in the sputum eosinophil count or FeNO is considered an indicator [16]. Patients with steroid-resistant asthma do not respond well to glucocorticosteroids and are mostly adults. Their FEV1 is considerably lower, with more air trapping, and there is an increased association with respiratory infections, obesity, smoking, and air pollution [8]. Increased sputum neutrophil counts and IL-17 levels can be used as biomarkers [7, 8]. Obesity-related asthma is thought to occur because of high-fat diet-related systemic inflammation, and L-arginine and leptin can be used as biomarkers [12]. Premenstrual or catamenial asthma is characterized by the deterioration of asthma symptoms in the premenstrual phase, and the role of hormone levels and systemic inflammation in these patients remains unknown [1]. Asthma in cross-country skiers or cold-induced asthma is characterized by mild to moderate symptoms and often triggered by exercise and cold. It is also associated with respiratory tract infection [14, 17]. Increased leukotriene (LT) E4 in urine may be used as a biomarker [14]. Exercise-induced asthma develops because of increased catecholamines during exercise, resulting in increased airway resistance [17]. Histamine and prostaglandin release reportedly play a role [17], but there is no specific biomarker. In asthma induced by stress or psychological factors, central nervous system activation by psychological stress, followed by the release of stress hormones (glucocorticoids, epinephrine, and norepinephrine) and immunological changes, may cause asthma exacerbation [18]. Although there is evidence regarding the critical role of psychological stress in the development and exacerbation of allergic asthma, this phenotype requires further research [18].

3. Asthma treatment and targets for biological drugs

A personalized approach with specific and targeted therapies for the cytokines constituting the inflammation cascade are of great benefit in the treatment of asthma, particularly the difficult-to-treat phenotypes [1, 14]. The pathophysiology of asthma has conventionally been mediated by Th2 lymphocytes, which induce the stimulation of eosinophils by IL-3, IL-5, and granulocyte–macrophage colony-stimulating factor (GM-CSF); basophils by IL-3; and mast cells by IL-4 and IL-9; alternatively, they cause direct mucosal damage via IL-4/IL-13 after antigen presentation [7–9]. Both IL-4 and IL-13 play a role in the activation of eosinophils, IgE synthesis, and, consequently, mucus secretion and airway remodeling [10]. However, they share the same receptor and signal pathways. All these cytokines also stimulate B-cells, causing the release of IgE. Currently approved targets for BD treatment in asthma include IgE, IL-4/IL-13, and IL-5, with uncontrolled or difficult-to-treat asthma requiring step 4 treatment as per the GINA guideline being the main indication [1]. In this group of patients, symptom control cannot be achieved despite maximum treatment [long-acting beta agonists (LABAs), tiotropium, high-dose ICSs, leukotriene antagonists, or theophylline with OCSs].

4. Classification for biologics

Biologics are divided into three common classes: monoclonal antibodies (mAbs), fusion proteins, and cytokines [2]. These drugs may be fully humanized mAbs or chimeric (human + murine mix) or fully murine/mouse antibodies [2, 19]. Diverse side effects with varying severities have been reported according to the level of humanization [3, 19]. Widely accepted nomenclature systems for biologics include the

USAN (the United States' Adopted Names) and INN (World Health Organization's International Nonproprietary Names) [2, 20]. Currently approved mAbs target IgE antibodies, cell surface molecules, soluble mediators, cytokines, viral proteins, and tumor antigens [2, 20]. Examples of these drugs include omalizumab (anti-IgE), rituximab (anti-CD20), infliximab [anti-tumor necrosis factor alpha (TNFα)], mepolizumab (anti-IL-5), and cetuximab (anti-epidermal growth factor receptor). Examples for fusion proteins; etanercept (anti-TNFα-RII), anakinra (anti-IL-1 receptor), and ritanercept (anti-IL-1β) are examples. The cytokine group includes recombinant cytokines such as interferon-α, interferon-β, GM-CSF, and IL-2.

5. Overview of biologics used for asthma treatment

Biologics have been used for the treatment of asthma since 2003. In the United States, omalizumab was the first drug approved for the treatment of severe and uncontrolled asthma [20]. Subsequently, several drugs targeting IgE, IL-5, IL-4, IL-5, IL-9, IL-13, IL-17, and TSLP were developed for the treatment of this patient group (**Table 3**). Details about these drugs are provided below.

5.1 Anti-IgE

a. **Omalizumab** (Xolair®) is a humanized mAb and the first drug to be approved by the Food and Drug Administration (FDA) for the treatment of severe uncontrolled asthma [21]. The mechanism of action involves selective binding to IgE antibodies, reduction of free IgE levels, and inhibition of inflammatory mediator release via the inhibition of mast cell degranulation.

   The PERSIST study, a "real-life" study, demonstrated that 12-month treatment with omalizumab can significantly improve the lung function and quality of life and minimize the rate of exacerbation [22]. The APEX II multicenter observational study demonstrated a clinical response rate to omalizumab at week 16 to be 82.4%. [23]. When the pre- and post-treatment periods were compared, a decrease in the daily OCS dose and number of exacerbations requiring hospitalization was observed. Moreover, pulmonary function test findings and the quality of life of patients were significantly improved. In a newly published study by Vennera et al., 60% patients who received omalizumab treatment for 6 years showed that the drug maintained its positive effect for at least 4 years after treatment discontinuation [24]. On the basis of clinical evidence, the response to omalizumab treatment is routinely evaluated after 16 weeks of treatment [25]; this evaluation is accepted as the most meaningful measurement and indication of permanent treatment response in the world.

   In pre- and postmarketing studies, the risk of anaphylaxis was reported to be 0.1%--0.2% [26]. It was found that 61% reactions occurred within 2 h after one of the first three doses, while 14% occurred within 30 min after a fourth or subsequent dose [27]. In another study, 3.4%, 2.2%, and 0% participants reported injection site reactions, hypersensitivity reactions (HSR), and anaphylaxis, respectively [28].

b. **Quilizumab** is a humanized mAb against the M1 major segment of membrane-bound IgE, and it causes memory depletion of B-cells and inhibits IgE production [29]. The primary indication is uncontrolled allergic asthma and chronic spontaneous urticaria. In a study by Harris et al., it was demonstrated that

Target	Generic Name	Brands	Release Status in EU
IgE	Omalizumab	Xolair®	12/2005, approved
	Quilizumab	-	Phase III
	Ligelizumab	-	Phase III
IL-5	Mepolizumab	Nucala®	12/2015, approved
	Reslizumab	Cinqaero®	08/2016, approved
IL-5R	Benralizumab	Fasenra®	01/2018, approved
IL-4R complex (IL-4/13)	Pitrakinra	Aerovant®	Phase IIb
	Dupilumab	Dupixent®	09/2018 approved
IL-13	Lebrikizumab	-	Stopped
	Tralokinumab	-	Stopped
IL-17A	Brodalumab	Kyntheum	Stopped
	Secukinumab	Cosentyx®	Phase II
IL-9	Enokizumab	—	Stopped
TSLP	Tezepelumab	—	Phase III
PG DP_2-receptor	Fevipiprant	QAW039	Phase III
	Timapiprant	OC-459	Phase II
	Setipipitrant	ACT-129968	Stopped

IgE,Immunglobulin E; IL, Interleukin; TSLP, thymic stromal lymphopoietin; EU, europa; FDA, Food and Drug Administration.

Table 3.
Overview of biological agents used in asthma.

quilizumab was well tolerated by patients and reduced the IgE levels (serum total and allergen-specific) by 30–40% [30]. However, there was no beneficial effect with regard to asthma exacerbations, lung function, and patient-reported symptom measures. At 36 weeks, the asthma exacerbation rate decreased by 19.6% relative to that in the placebo group, although this was not a statistically significant result. Significant clinical efficacy benefit has not been demonstrated in studies of various biomarker subgroups (serum IgE, blood eosinophils, exhaled NO, and periostin). The safety of the drug was evaluated in the same study, and injection site reactions (mostly pain) were reported in 6.9% patients [30]. Currently, phase III studies of this drug are in progress.

c. **Ligelizumab** is an investigational humanized mAb that binds to IgE with a higher affinity than does omalizumab. In a 2016 study of patients with mild allergic asthma, it was found that inhaled and skin allergen responses were 3-fold and 16-fold greater with ligelizumab than with omalizumab and placebo, respectively [31]. These findings suggest the effectiveness of this drug in asthma treatment; phase III studies are currently ongoing.

5.2 Anti-IL-5

a. **Mepolizumab** (Nucala®) is a humanized mAb that binds to IL-5, selectively inhibits eosinophilic inflammation, and reduces both sputum and the number of eosinophils in the blood [32]. After receiving approval for the treatment of eosinophilic and severe asthma in Europe in December 2015, it was approved for the treatment of eosinophilic granulomatosis with polyangiitis and Churg–Strauss syndrome in December 2017.

In one study, subcutaneous administration of mepolizumab 100 mg every 4 days significantly lowered the rate of asthma exacerbations and the daily dose of OCSs in patients dependent on OCSs for asthma control [33]. In another study, mepolizumab was found to be at least as effective as omalizumab, and no significant difference was found between the tolerability profiles of the two treatments [34]. The most commonly reported adverse events in the Dose Ranging Efficiency and Safety with Mepolizumab in Severe Asthma (DREAM) study were nonallergic reactions associated with infusion [35]. In addition, Lugogo et al. [36] observed HSRs in <1% patients, injection site reactions in 4%, and infusion/injection reactions (nonallergic) in 1%. None of the recent studies has reported the occurrence of anaphylaxis as a side effect [35, 36].

b. **Reslizumab** (Cinqaero®) is a humanized mAb that binds to IL-5 and is used as an adjunctive drug in the treatment of severe and uncontrolled eosinophilic asthma [37]. The drug inhibits the activation, differentiation, and growth of eosinophils by inhibiting the binding of IL-5 to eosinophils. Unlike other drugs, it is intravenously administered at a dose of 3 mg/kg every 4 weeks.

In a subgroup analysis by Corren et al., the efficacy of resolizumab for an improvement in respiratory function, Asthma Control Questionnaire (ACQ) scores, and recovery inhaler use were evaluated for patients with a blood eosinophil count of >400 cells/μL [38]. Therefore, the blood eosinophil count is a useful pre-treatment biomarker in predicting patients' response to therapy and for the appropriate patient selection. In addition, two phase III studies reported that reslizumab administration improves lung function and controls asthma and related symptoms in patients with severe, uncontrolled, eosinophilic (≥400 cells/μL) asthma [38, 39]. Murphy et al. [40] demonstrated the long-term clinical effects and reported HSRs (<1%), drug rash (<1%), and very rare local infusion-related adverse events (e.g., pain at the site of injection; <1%) during the follow-up period, with no documented case of anaphylaxis [40].

c. **Benralizumab** (Fasenra®) is the newest biologics in the family of humanized mAbs, and it is being developed for the treatment of eosinophilic and allergic asthma [41]. Its acts by binding to the α-subunit of the IL-5 receptor (IL5Rα) on eosinophils and basophils.

In the SIROCCO [42] and CALIMA [43] trials, both phase III trials, benralizumab significantly lowered the annual exacerbation rate in patients with uncontrolled asthma (despite high-dose ICS plus LABA treatment) and a blood eosinophil count of >300 cells/μL. The safety of the drug was also tested, and it was found to be well tolerated. Following these promising data, it was approved for use in Europe in the beginning of 2018. The most commonly reported side effect is mild to moderate nasopharyngitis [44]. FDA labels report a HSR (rash, urticaria) rate of 3% for patients receiving benralizumab and placebo therapy [41]. In these labels, the rate of injection site reactions was 2.2% for patients treated with benralizumab and 1.9% for those treated with placebo, with two cases of anaphylaxis [41]. Post-marketing recording and notification of side effects are currently ongoing.

5.3 Anti-IL-4/13

a. **Pitrakinra:** (Aerovant®) is a human recombinant protein that competitively inhibits the IL-4Ra complex, thus showing antagonism to IL-4 and IL-13 [45]. In phase II studies, FEV1 was measured 4–10 h after an allergen challenge in patients with atopic asthma (46), and patients treated with pitrakinra showed a lesser decrease in FEV1 than did those treated with placebo [46]. Moreover, improvements in pulmonary function test findings, decreased exhaled nitric oxide levels, and decreased allergic responses were reported [46]. Phase IIb studies of this drug, which can be taken via a dry-powder inhaler or subcutaneously, are ongoing [45].

b. **Dupilumab** (Dupixent®) is a fully human mAb that can be subcutaneously administered. It binds to the IL-4Ra complex (also inhibits the effects of both IL-4 and IL-13) [47]. In a recent randomized, double-blind, phase III study, subcutaneous administration of dupilumab 200–300 mg (once every two weeks) significantly decreased the asthma exacerbation rate in patients with severe uncontrolled asthma and type 2 inflammation [47]. In another study, placebo and dupilumab showed no significant differences in the rate of mild and severe adverse events, death, drug discontinuation due to side effects, and incidence of upper respiratory tract infections, influenza, and bronchitis [48]. However, dupilumab was associated with an increased risk of injection site reactions [48]. This BD has been approved for use in the treatment of atopic dermatitis, and its use for severe asthma was approved by the FDA in 2018.

5.4 Anti-IL-13

a. **Lebrikizumab** is a new humanized IgG4 mAb that can be subcutaneously administered. It specifically inhibits IL-13 activity [49]. This drug was administered to patients with uncontrolled asthma, and FENO significantly decreased in the high periostin group (4.3%) compared with that in the low periostin group (34.4%) [49]. In a phase III study of the drug, no clinically meaningful decrease in the asthma exacerbation rate could be found in patients with high biomarker levels (periostin ≥50 ng/mL or blood eosinophils ≥300 cells/μL) [50]. Moreover, in a study by Korenblat et al., 12 weeks of treatment for patients with mild-to-moderate asthma did not result in adequate improvements in the results of prebronchodilator lung function tests [51].

b. **Tralokinumab** is a mAb that acts on IL-13, which is still being studied today. The results of a previous study revealed that, despite a consistent improvement in FEV1 in the FENO-high group, there was no possibility of a significant clinical benefit in patients with severe uncontrolled asthma [52]. A promising biomarker to predict the responsiveness to anti-IL-13 treatment has been found, and further studies are underway [53]. It is necessary to investigate the effects of this drug on different asthma phenotypes.

5.5 Anti-IL-17

Secukinumab and Brodalumab are monoclonal antibodies that target IL-17A and IL-17RA signaling, respectively. A phase II trial of the efficacy and safety of secukinumab treatment for asthma has been completed (NCT01478360), and the results are expected. On the other hand, a phase II trial of brodalumab (NCT01902290) was terminated because of the lack of efficacy in a predetermined intermediate analysis. Both drugs are approved and presently used for the treatment of moderate to severe plaque psoriasis.

5.6 Anti-IL-9

Enokizumab (Medi-528), which is a mAb against IL-9, is defined as a T-cell and mast cell growth factor [54]. It was initially tested in animal models of asthma and was shown to alleviate the disease [54]. Subsequently, a double-blind, multicenter study involving 329 human adults was conducted [55], and the results revealed that the addition of this drug to existing anti-asthma drugs does not improve FEV1 values, decrease the asthma exacerbation rate, or improve ACQ scores. This observation was surprising, considering the very promising initial results. The main reason for this discrepancy is thought to be the heterogeneity of the study patients and the lack of differentiation between asthma subtypes [55].

5.7 Anti-epithelial cell-derived cytokine

Tezepelumab is a human mAb specific for TSLP, which is an epithelial cytokine. TSLP is considered to play a critical role in the onset and progress of airway inflammation. In a study by Corren et al., 52-week treatment with this BD significantly decreased the asthma exacerbation rate, independent of the blood eosinophil count [56]. Moreover, the prebronchodilator FEV1 at 52 weeks was higher in all tezepelumab groups than in the placebo group (mean, 110–150 mL) [56]. This is a very promising drug for noneosinophilic, uncontrolled asthma, and phase III studies (NCT03927157, and NCT03347279) are currently ongoing.

5.8 Prostoglandin DP2 receptor antagonist

Fevipiprant and Timapiprant is a promising biologics has been set for new biological treatments in allergic asthma. This target is prostaglandin D2 (PGD2) which acts through the DP2 receptor, also known as chemoattractant receptor-homologous molecule expressed on Th2 cells (CRTh2). DP2 is a G-protein-dependent receptor that mediates activation and migration of Th2 cells and eosinophils at the center of allergic and inflammatory processes.

Fevipiprant is a powerful, reversible and highly selective DP2 receptor antagonist that can be used orally, targeting PGD2 directly [57]. In phase 2 studies performed in patients with severe uncontrolled eosinophilic asthma, the rate of sputum eosinophils decreased, 160–207 ml increase in FEV1 level and Asthma Control Questionnaire scores was obtained [58]. Phase III studies (NCT02555683 and NCT02563067) was completed and the results are expected. If positive results are obtained in these studies, it can be thought that this oral treatment would be an alternative to the biological treatments and would be easier to access.

Timapiprant (OC000459), which also affected the same receptor, showed 95 ml FEV1 increase in mild to moderate allergic asthma compared to placebo, and in the post hoc analysis, 220 ml increase was reported in FEV1 compared to placebo when atopic eosinophilic uncontrolled asthma subjects were selected [59]. No serious drug-related side effects were reported in the same study.

6. Conclusion

In summary, BDs play an important role in the treatment of many lung diseases. Recent advances in our knowledge of asthma pathologies, the role of cytokines, allergen-directed immune responses, and disease phenotyping have resulted in the identification of numerous potential and specific targets for BDs. Monoclonal antibodies targeting IgE, IL-5 and IL-4/IL-13 have demonstrated significant improvements in asthma control such as reduce asthma exacerbations and improve lung functions [60]. In addition, long-term benefits such as reduced need for oral corticosteroids and control medications, reduction in asthma symptoms, improving quality of life, and reduced loss of work capacity have been demonstrated [7–9]. For the future, there is a need for new biomarkers to identify asthma patients with Th2-low endotype and thus new BDs that affect inflammatory pathways [60].

On the other hand, anti-IL-9 and anti-IL-17 treatments showed no positive results in terms of clinical benefits [55]. Meanwhile, anti-TSLP and anti-PGD2 treatment has shown very promising results, and the results of phase III studies are awaited. However, because of the increasing number of BDs and associated studies, it has become very difficult to update treatment guidelines on a regular basis; this issue and personalized treatment options needs to be resolved in future. However, after the endotypes and phenotypes are classified, investigation of the effects of these drugs may yield different results.

Conflict of interest

The authors declare no conflict of interest.

Author details

Aşkın Gülşen
Department of Pneumology, University of Lübeck, Germany

*Address all correspondence to: askingulsen@hotmail.com

References

[1] Global Strategy for Asthma Management and Prevention. https://ginasthma.org (accessed on 02 Januar 2021).

[2] World Health Organization. International Nonproprietary Names (INN) for Biological and Biotechnological Substances. (A Review) - Update 2016. https://www.who.int/medicines/services/inn/BioReview2016.pdf (accessed on 02 Januar 2021).

[3] Gülsen A, Wedi B, Jappe U. Hypersensitivity reactions to biologics (part I): allergy as an important differential diagnosis in complex immune-derived adverse events. Allergo J. 2020;29:32-61. German. DOI: 10.1007/s15007-020-2550-1.

[4] Simpson JL, Scott R, Boyle MJ, Gibson PG. Inflammatory subtypes in asthma: assessment and identification using induced sputum. Respirology. 2006;11:54-61. DOI: 10.1111/j.1440-1843.2006.00784.x.

[5] Moore WC, Meyers DA, Wenzel SE, Teague WG, Li H, Li X, et al; National Heart, Lung, and Blood Institute's Severe Asthma Research Program. Identification of asthma phenotypes using cluster analysis in the Severe Asthma Research Program. Am J Respir Crit Care Med. 2010;181:315-323. DOI: 10.1164/rccm.200906-0896OC.

[6] Moore WC, Hastie AT, Li X, Li H, Busse WW, Jarjour NN, et al; National Heart, Lung, and Blood Institute's Severe Asthma Research Program. Sputum neutrophil counts are associated with more severe asthma phenotypes using cluster analysis. J Allergy Clin Immunol. 2014;133:1557-1563. DOI: 10.1016/j.jaci.2013.10.011

[7] Skloot GS. Asthma phenotypes and endotypes: a personalized approach to treatment. Curr Opin Pulm Med. 2016;22:3-9. DOI: 10.1097/MCP.0000000000000225.

[8] Godar M, Blanchetot C, de Haard H, Lambrecht BN, Brusselle G. Personalized medicine with biologics for severe type 2 asthma: current status and future prospects. MAbs. 2018;10:34-45. DOI: 10.1080/19420862.2017.1392425.

[9] Braido F, Tiotiu A, Kowal K, Mihaicuta S, Novakova P, Oguzulgen IK. Phenotypes/endotypes-driven treatment in asthma. Curr Opin Allergy Clin Immunol. 2018;18:184-189. DOI: 10.1097/ACI.0000000000000440.

[10] Stokes JR, Casale TB. Characterization of asthma endotypes: implications for therapy. Ann Allergy Asthma Immunol. 2016;117:121-125. DOI: 10.1016/j.anai.2016.05.016.

[11] Yan X, Chu JH, Gomez J, Koenigs M, Holm C, He X,et al. Noninvasive Analysis of the Sputum Transcriptome Discriminates Clinical Phenotypes of Asthma. Ann Am Thorac Soc. 2016;13 Suppl 1:S104-5. DOI: 10.1513/AnnalsATS.201510-681MG.

[12] Ilmarinen P, Tuomisto LE, Kankaanranta H. Phenotypes, Risk Factors, and Mechanisms of Adult-Onset Asthma. Mediators Inflamm. 2015;2015:514868. DOI: 10.1155/2015/514868.

[13] Pembrey L, Barreto ML, Douwes J, Cooper P, Henderson J, Mpairwe H, Ardura-Garcia C, Chico M, Brooks C, Cruz AA, Elliott AM, Figueiredo CA, Langan SM, Nassanga B, Ring S, Rodrigues L, Pearce N. Understanding asthma phenotypes: the World Asthma Phenotypes (WASP) international collaboration. ERJ Open Res. 2018;4:13. DOI: 10.1183/23120541.00013-2018.

[14] Lötvall J, Akdis CA, Bacharier LB, Bjermer L, Casale TB, Custovic A, et al.

Asthma endotypes: a new approach to classification of disease entities within the asthma syndrome. J Allergy Clin Immunol. 2011;127:355-360. DOI: 10.1016/j.jaci.2010.11.037.

[15] Muñoz X, Cruz MJ, Bustamante V, Lopez-Campos JL, Barreiro E. Work-related asthma: diagnosis and prognosis of immunological occupational asthma and work-exacerbated asthma. J Investig Allergol Clin Immunol. 2014;24:396-405. PMID: 25668891.

[16] Hirose M, Horiguchi T. Asthma phenotypes. J Gen Fam Med. 2017;18:189-194. DOI: 10.1002/jgf2.7.

[17] Giesbrecht GG, Younes M. Exercise- and cold-induced asthma. Can J Appl Physiol. 1995;20:300-314. DOI: 10.1139/h95-023.

[18] Ohno I. Neuropsychiatry phenotype in asthma: Psychological stress-induced alterations of the neuroendocrine-immune system in allergic airway inflammation. Allergol Int. 2017;66S: S2-S8. DOI: 10.1016/j.alit.2017.06.005.

[19] Hwang WY, Foote J. Immunogenicity of engineered antibodies. Methods. 2005;36:3-10. DOI: 10.1016/j.ymeth.2005.01.001.

[20] American Medical Association. AMA (USAN) Monoclonal antibodies. *United States Adopted Names.* https://www.ama-assn.org/about/monoclonal-antibodies (accessed on 02 Januar 2021).

[21] U.S. Food and Drug Administration, Omalizumab https://www.accessdata.fda.gov/drugsatfda_docs/label/2016/103976s5225lbl.pdf (accessed on 02 Januar 2021).

[22] Brusselle G, Michils A, Louis R, Dupont L, Van de Maele B, Delobbe A, et. al. "Real-life" effectiveness of omalizumab in patients with severe persistent allergic asthma: The PERSIST study. Respir Med. 2009;103:1633-1642. DOI: 10.1016/j.rmed.2009.06.014.

[23] Niven RM, Saralaya D, Chaudhuri R, Masoli M, Clifton I, Mansur AH, et al. Impact of omalizumab on treatment of severe allergic asthma in UK clinical practice: a UK multicentre observational study (the APEX II study). BMJ Open. 2016;6:e011857. DOI:10.1136/bmjopen-2016-011857.

[24] Vennera MDC, Sabadell C, Picado C; Spanish Omalizumab Registry. Duration of the efficacy of omalizumab after treatment discontinuation in 'real life' severe asthma. Thorax. 2018;73:782-784. DOI: 10.1136/thoraxjnl-2017-210017.

[25] Lin CH, Cheng SL. A review of omalizumab for the management of severe asthma. Drug Des Devel Ther. 2016;10:2369-2378. DOI: 10.2147/DDDT.S112208.

[26] Baker DL, Nakamura GR, Lowman HB, Fischer SK. Evaluation of IgE Antibodies to Omalizumab (Xolair®) and Their Potential Correlation to Anaphylaxis. *AAPS J*. 2015;18:115-123. DOI: 10.1208/s12248-015-9821-x.

[27] Cox L, Platts-Mills TA, Finegold I, Schwartz LB, Simons FE, Wallace DV; American Academy of Allergy, Asthma & Immunology; American College of Allergy, Asthma and Immunology. American Academy of Allergy, Asthma & Immunology/American College of Allergy, Asthma and Immunology Joint Task Force Report on omalizumab-associated anaphylaxis. J Allergy Clin Immunol. 2007;120:1373-1377. DOI: 10.1016/j.jaci.2007.09.032.

[28] Di Bona D, Fiorino I, Taurino M, Frisenda F, Minenna E, Pasculli C,et al. Long-term "real-life" safety of omalizumab in patients with severe uncontrolled asthma: A nine-year study. Respir Med. 2017;130:55-60. DOI: 10.1016/j.rmed.2017.07.013.

[29] Brightbill HD, Jeet S, Lin Z, Yan D, Zhou M, Tan M, Nguyen et al. Antibodies specific for a segment of

human membrane IgE deplete IgE-producing B cells in humanized mice. J Clin Invest. 2010;120:2218-2229. DOI: 10.1172/JCI40141.

[30] Harris JM, Maciuca R, Bradley MS, Cabanski CR, Scheerens H, Lim J, Cai F, Kishnani M, Liao XC, Samineni D, Zhu R, Cochran C, Soong W, Diaz JD, Perin P, Tsukayama M, Dimov D, Agache I, Kelsen SG. A randomized trial of the efficacy and safety of quilizumab in adults with inadequately controlled allergic asthma. Respir Res. 2016;17:29. DOI: 10.1186/s12931-016-0347-2.

[31] Gauvreau GM, Arm JP, Boulet LP, Leigh R, Cockcroft DW, Davis BE, et al. Efficacy and safety of multiple doses of QGE031 (ligelizumab) versus omalizumab and placebo in inhibiting allergen-induced early asthmatic responses. J Allergy Clin Immunol. 2016;138:1051-1059. DOI: 10.1016/j.jaci.2016.02.027.

[32] Ortega HG, Liu MC, Pavord ID, Brusselle GG, FitzGerald JM, Chetta A, et al; MENSA Investigators. Mepolizumab treatment in patients with severe eosinophilic asthma. N Engl J Med. 2014;371:1198-1207. DOI: 10.1056/NEJMoa1403290.

[33] Deeks ED. Mepolizumab: A Review in Eosinophilic Asthma. BioDrugs. 2016;30:361-370. DOI: 10.1007/s40259-016-0182-5.

[34] Cockle SM, Stynes G, Gunsoy NB, Parks D, Alfonso-Cristancho R, Wex J, Bradford ES, Albers FC, Willson J. Comparative effectiveness of mepolizumab and omalizumab in severe asthma: An indirect treatment comparison. Respir Med. 2017;123:140-148. DOI: 10.1016/j.rmed.2016.12.009.

[35] Pavord ID, Korn S, Howarth P, Bleecker ER, Buhl R, Keene ON, Ortega H, Chanez P. Mepolizumab for severe eosinophilic asthma (DREAM): a multicentre, double-blind, placebo-controlled trial. Lancet (London, England). 2012;380:651-659. DOI: 10.1016/S0140-6736(12)60988-X.

[36] Lugogo N, Domingo C, Chanez P, Leigh R, Gilson MJ, Price RG, et al. Long-term efficacy and safety of mepolizumab in patients with severe eosinophilic asthma: a multi-center, open-label, Phase IIIb study. Clin Ther. 2016:1-14. DOI: 10.1016/j.clinthera.2016.07.010.

[37] Máspero J. Reslizumab in the treatment of inadequately controlled asthma in adults and adolescents with elevated blood eosinophils: clinical trial evidence and future prospects. Ther Adv Respir Dis. 2017;11:311-325. DOI: 10.1177/1753465817717134.

[38] Corren J, Weinstein S, Janka L, Zangrilli J, Garin M. Phase 3 Study of Reslizumab in Patients With Poorly Controlled Asthma: Effects Across a Broad Range of Eosinophil Counts. Chest. 2016;150:799-810. DOI: 10.1016/j.chest.2016.03.018.

[39] Bjermer L, Lemiere C, Maspero J, Weiss S, Zangrilli J, Germinaro M. Reslizumab for Inadequately Controlled Asthma With Elevated Blood Eosinophil Levels: A Randomized Phase 3 Study. Chest. 2016;150:789-798. DOI: 10.1016/j.chest.2016.03.032

[40] Murphy K, Jacobs J, Bjermer L, Fahrenholz JM, Shalit Y, Garin M, et al. Long-term Safety and Efficacy of Reslizumab in Patients with Eosinophilic Asthma. J Allergy Clin Immunol Pract. 2017;5:1572-1581. DOI: 10.1016/j.jaip.2017.08.024.

[41] US Food and Drug Administration. FDA labels for Benralizumab. https://www.accessdata.fda.gov/drugsatfda_docs/nda/2017/761070Orig1s000SumR.pdf (websites accessed 05 November 2018)

[42] Bleecker ER, FitzGerald JM, Chanez P, Papi A, Weinstein SF,

Barker P, et al; SIROCCO study investigators. Efficacy and safety of benralizumab for patients with severe asthma uncontrolled with high-dosage inhaled corticosteroids and long-acting β(2)-agonists (SIROCCO): a randomised, multicentre, placebo-controlled phase 3 trial. Lancet. 2016;388:2115-2127. DOI: 10.1016/S0140-6736(16)31324-1.

[43] FitzGerald JM, Bleecker ER, Nair P, Korn S, Ohta K, Lommatzsch M, et al. Benralizumab, an anti-interleukin-5 receptor α monoclonal antibody, as add-on treatment for patients with severe, uncontrolled, eosinophilic asthma (CALIMA): a randomised, double-blind, placebo-controlled phase 3 trial. Lancet. 2016;388:2128-2141. DOI: 10.1016/S0140-6736(16)31322-8.

[44] Khorasanizadeh M, Eskian M, Assa'ad AH, Camargo CA Jr, Rezaei N. Efficacy and Safety of Benralizumab, a Monoclonal Antibody against IL-5Rα,in Uncontrolled Eosinophilic Asthma. Int Rev Immunol. 2016;35:294-311. DOI: 10.3109/08830185.2015.1128901.

[45] Long AA. Monoclonal antibodies and other biologic agents in the treatment of asthma. MAbs. 2009;1:237-246. DOI: 10.4161/mabs.1.3.8352.

[46] Wenzel S, Wilbraham D, Fuller R, Getz EB, Longphre M. Effect of an interleukin-4 variant on late phase asthmatic response to allergen challenge in asthmatic patients: results of two phase 2a studies. Lancet. 2007;370:1422-1231. DOI: 10.1016/S0140-6736(07)61600-6.

[47] Busse WW, Maspero JF, Rabe KF, Papi A, Wenzel SE, Ford LB, Pavord ID, Zhang B, Staudinger H, Pirozzi G, Amin N, Akinlade B, Eckert L, Chao J, Graham NMH, Teper A. Liberty Asthma QUEST: Phase 3 Randomized, Double-Blind, Placebo-Controlled, Parallel-Group Study to Evaluate Dupilumab Efficacy/Safety in Patients with Uncontrolled, Moderate-to-Severe Asthma. Adv Ther. 2018;35:737-748. DOI: 10.1007/s12325-018-0702-4.

[48] Zayed Y, Kheiri B, Banifadel M, Hicks M, Aburahma A, Hamid K, Bachuwa G,Chandran A. Dupilumab safety and efficacy in uncontrolled asthma: a systematic review and meta-analysis of randomized clinical trials. J Asthma. 2018:1-10. DOI: 10.1080/02770903.2018.1520865.

[49] Agrawal S, Townley RG. Role of periostin, FENO, IL-13, lebrikzumab, other IL-13 antagonist and dual IL-4/IL-13 antagonist in asthma. Expert Opin Biol Ther. 2014;14:165-181. DOI: 10.1517/14712598.2014.859673.

[50] Hanania NA, Korenblat P, Chapman KR, Bateman ED, Kopecky P, Paggiaro P, et al. Efficacy and safety of lebrikizumab in patients with uncontrolled asthma (LAVOLTA I and LAVOLTA II): replicate, phase 3, randomised, double-blind, placebo-controlled trials. Lancet Respir Med. 2016;4:781-796. DOI: 10.1016/S2213-2600(16)30265-X.

[51] Korenblat P, Kerwin E, Leshchenko I, Yen K, Holweg CTJ, Anzures-Cabrera J,Martin C, Putnam WS, Governale L, Olsson J, Matthews JG. Efficacy and safety oflebrikizumab in adult patients with mild-to-moderate asthma not receiving inhaled corticosteroids. Respir Med. 2018;134:143-149. DOI: 10.1016/j.rmed.2017.12.006.

[52] Chung KF. Tralokinumab unsuccessful for management of severe, uncontrolled asthma. Lancet Respir Med. 2018;6:480-481. DOI: 10.1016/S2213-2600(18)30194-2.

[53] Nakamura Y, Sugano A, Ohta M, Takaoka Y. Docking analysis and the possibilityof prediction efficacy for an anti-IL-13 biopharmaceutical treatment with tralokinumab and lebrikizumab for bronchial asthma. PLoS One.

2017;12:e0188407. DOI: 10.1371/journal.pone.0188407.

[54] Gong F, Pan YH, Huang X, Zhu HY, Jiang DL. From bench to bedside: Therapeuticpotential of interleukin-9 in the treatment of asthma. Exp Ther Med. 2017;13:389-394. DOI: 10.3892/etm.2017.4024.

[55] Oh CK, Leigh R, McLaurin KK, Kim K, Hultquist M, Molfino NA. A randomized,controlled trial to evaluate the effect of an anti-interleukin-9 monoclonal antibody in adults with uncontrolled asthma. Respir Res. 2013;14:93. DOI: 10.1186/1465-9921-14-93.

[56] Corren J, Parnes JR, Wang L, Mo M, Roseti SL, Griffiths JM, et al. Tezepelumab in Adults with Uncontrolled Asthma. N Engl J Med. 2017;377:936-946. DOI: 10.1056/NEJMoa1704064.

[57] Luu VT, Goujon JY, Meisterhans C, Frommherz M, Bauer C. Synthesis of a high specific activity methyl sulfone tritium isotopologue of fevipiprant (NVP-QAW039). J Labelled Comp Radiopharm. 2015;58:188-195. DOI: 10.1002/jlcr.3281.

[58] Murillo JC, Dimov V, Gonzalez-Estrada A. An evaluation of fevipiprant for the treatment of asthma: a promising new therapy? Expert Opin Pharmacother. 2018:1-7. DOI: 10.1080/14656566.2018.1540589.

[59] Pettipher R, Hunter MG, Perkins CM, Collins LP, Lewis T, Baillet M, et al. Heightened response of eosinophilic asthmatic patients to the CRTH2 antagonist OC000459. Allergy. 2014;69:1223-1232. DOI: 10.1111/all.12451.

[60] McGregor MC, Krings JG, Nair P, Castro M. Role of Biologics in Asthma. Am J Respir Crit Care Med. 2019;199:433-445. DOI: 10.1164/rccm.201810-1944CI.

Chapter 6

Anaphylactic Reactions in Radiology Procedures

Callen Kwamboka Onyambu, Angeline Anyona Aywak, Sarah Kemunto Osiemo and Timothy Musila Mutala

Abstract

Reactions to contrast agents are uncommon but range from mild urticaria to life threatening anaphylactic reactions. Majority of these reactions occur due to intravenous administration of iodinated contrast media. Acute reactions to MRI gadolinium-based contrast are much less common but they do occur and thus have to be managed. Usual presentations include urticaria, nausea, vomiting, angioedema, bronchospasm, laryngospasm and systemic hypotension. Majority of these reactions occur within the first twenty minutes after administration of contrast. Therefore, their recognition and prompt treatment are critical for good patient outcome. Attendant to this the radiology department must be adequately prepared to handle these emergencies as and when they do occur. This means an up to date emergency tray must be checked regularly before the start of the procedure, ensure there is epinephrine, antihistamines, beta-2-agonists metered dose inhalers, IV fluids, and ready supply of oxygen. Close collaboration of radiology staff with the hospital emergency response team is critical since severe reactions will need the intervention of this team.

Keywords: anaphylaxis, iodinated contrast, bronchospasm, hypotension, diagnosis, treatment

1. Introduction

Contrast media is a substance that is used to enhance the differentiation of tissues within the body in medical imaging. They are administered either intravenously, intraarterially, orally or into body cavities, majority being administered intravenously. Over the past few years there has been an increase in the number of radiographic examinations that use contrast media for better lesion characterization, more so in CT and MRI examinations [1]. Although contrast media has become progressively safer over time, especially with the use of low osmolar contrast media (LOCM), anaphylactic reactions still do occur. It is estimated that 0.6% of iodinated and 0.12% of gadolinium contrast cause anaphylactic reactions [2–4]. Reactions to contrast media range from mild reactions to life threatening severe reactions. Most acute reactions occur within 1 hour of contrast media administration, with majority occurring within the first 20 minutes. Therefore, it is important to be aware of these reactions, to monitor the patient closely in this period and to manage the reactions when they do occur [5].

There are two main types of iodinated contrast comprising high osmolar (HOCM) or ionic contrast that dissociates in solution to form particles and low

Types of contrast media				
Contrast	**Trade name**	**Ionic/Non-ionic**	**Iodine content**	**Osmolarity**
Diatrizoate	Gastrografin	Ionic	300mg/ml	1550
Ioxaglate	Hexabrix	Ionic	320mg/ml	580
Ultravist	Iopromide	Non-ionic	300mg/ml	607
Optiray	Ioversal	Non-ionic	300mg/ml	651
Isovue 370	Iopamidol	Non-ionic	370mg/ml	796
Omnipaque 300	Iohexol	Non-ionic	300mg/ml	672
Ioxilan 350	Oxilan	Non-ionic	350mg/ml	695
Iotrol 300	Iotrolan	Non-ionic	300mg/ml	310
Visipaque 320	Iodixanol	Non-ionic	320mg/ml	290

Table 1.
Types of iodine based contrast media and osmolarity.

osmolar or non-ionic that does not dissociate in solution. Contrast media osmolality is determined by the number of particles formed in solution. Ionic contrast media dissociates into osmotically active ions in solution and therefore have a higher osmolality. Non-ionic agents do not dissociate to ions when dissolved in solution and hence have a lower osmolality. In recent years there has been a shift to using the LOCM because of associated fewer reactions therefore making contrast administration safer. Nevertheless, acute anaphylactic reactions can still occur unpredictably and therefore must be recognized and managed promptly. Some of the commonly used iodine-based contrast agents and their osmolality are listed in **Table 1** above.

2. Gadolinium based contrast

Gadolinium based MRI contrast agents have been shown to be safe for intravenous administration, and actually a better safety profile than iodinated contrast for CT and other radiographic examinations. However acute reactions do occur and include urticaria, nausea and vomiting, and rarely anaphylaxis. In a study of 141,623 doses of MRI contrast administered Jae-woo et al. identified 0.079% immediate hypersensitivity reactions including urticaria, angioedema, bronchospasm and anaphylaxis and one fatality giving a mortality rate of 0.007% [6].

3. Presentation and management of contrast reactions

3.1 Clinical presentation

Reactions can be categorized as mild, moderate and severe as well as immediate and delayed. Mild reactions are usually self-limiting and require just supportive treatment, whereas moderate to severe reactions require prompt treatment. Delayed reactions such as abdominal pains, joint pains, fever and chills, diarrhea, headache, rashes and dizziness may be seen within two weeks from the date of contrast administration. Renal toxicity is also a commonly encountered side effect of contrast reactions manifesting as impaired renal function within two weeks of contrast administration.

Table 2 below shows the different types of reactions seen.

Severity	Reaction
Mild reactions	Urticaria
	Hives
	Nausea
	Vomiting
Moderate reactions	Facial oedema
	Severe vomiting
	Bronchospasm
	Laryngeal oedema
Severe reactions	Pulmonary oedema
	Cardiac arrythmia
	Cardiovascular collapse
	Respiratory collapse

Table 2.
Classification of contrast media reactions.

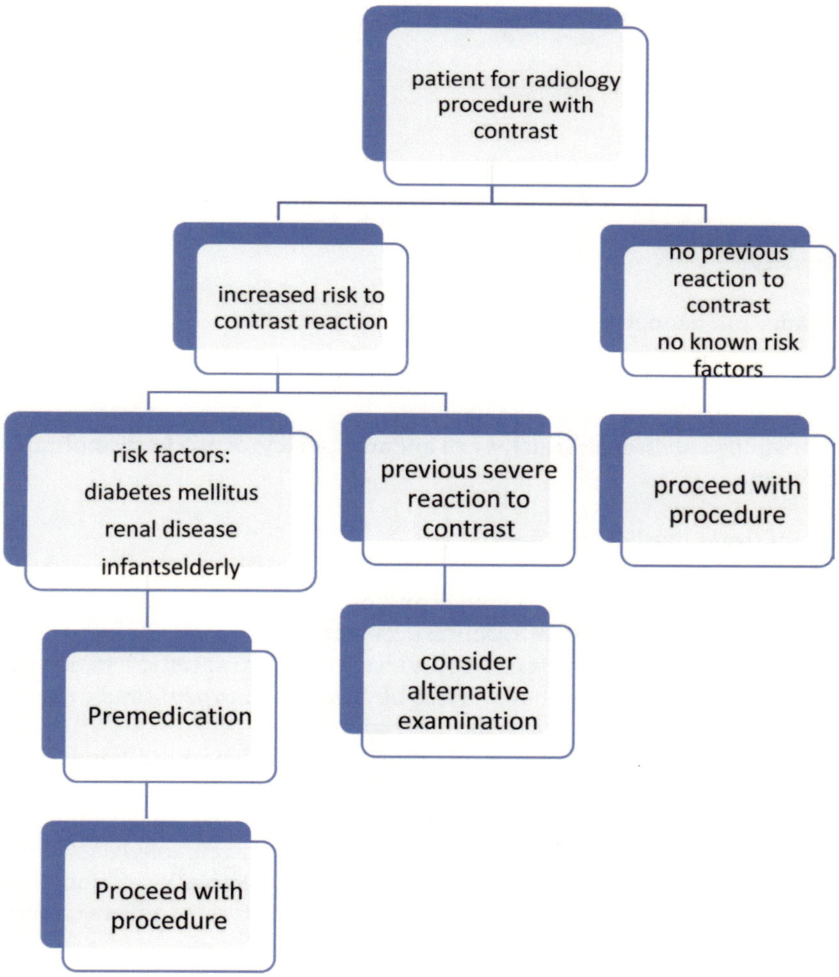

Figure 1.
Patient evaluation algorithm.

Anaphylactic reaction usually occurs within one hour of contrast administration, with majority occurring within the first 20 minutes. This is a life-threatening reaction and manifests with hypotension, bronchospasm/laryngeal oedema and circulatory collapse. Patient evaluation algorithm is as outlined in **Figure 1** above.

4. Anaphylactic reactions to contrast media

Although contrast side effects are infrequent, the knowledge of their presentation, their relationship with pre existing conditions and their management is required to ensure optimal patient care [2, 7]. Non ionic agents are iso-osmolar or low osmolar in nature and have fewer adverse effects [8, 9].

Majority of contrast reactions occur unpredictably and severe reactions may occur even when there has been a previous uneventful examination.

Risk factors that increase the likelihood of occurrence of adverse reactions [10–12] include:

1. Previous history of allergy like reaction to contrast media.
2. Allergy to food or other drugs.
3. History of asthma.
4. Renal insufficiency.
5. Cardiac disease e.g. Congestive cardiac failure, angina.
6. Anxiety.
7. Infants and neonates.
8. Elderly, above the age of 60 years.
9. Hematological disorders: sickle cell anemia, polycythemia vera, multiple myeloma.
10. Use of drugs like beta blockers.

A detailed history should be obtained and pre medication administered prior to contrast use to reduce the risk of reaction occurrence.

Adverse reactions to contrast can be divided into organ specific and non organ specific or general reactions. They can also be classified into acute and delayed based on the timing after contrast administration.

Acute hypersensitivity reactions are those that develop within 1 hour of contrast administration and can classified into allergic-like and physiologic [13]. Allergic-like reactions are largely dose and concentration independent. They do not require prior sensitization or Ig-E and are thus called idiosyncratic /anaphylactoid reactions. They occur via direct mast cell stimulations or via activation of complement by immune complexes [14]. These are the most frequent type of adverse reactions and may have serious, occasionally fatal, complications.

Physiologic reactions are those that are dose and concentration dependent are thus called non idiosyncratic reactions. They are due to direct chemotoxic or osmotoxic effects of the contrast media [15].

These acute reactions can be further subclassified into into 3 categories based on severity-mild, moderate and severe [11]. Mild reactions are those that are self limiting. The mild allergic-like reactions include limited urticaria, pruritus, cutaneous edema, nasal congestion while the physiologic reactions include limited nausea and vomiting, transient flushing, headache, dizziness, anxiety and vasovagal reactions that resolve spontaneously [16]. Moderate reactions are those that are progressive and more pronounced and require medical management [17, 18]. The moderate allergic-like reactions include diffuse urticaria/pruritus, diffuse erythema with normal vital signs, facial edema, throat tightness, wheezing and bronchospasms. While the moderate physiological reactions include protracted vomiting, hypertensive urgency, vasovagal reactions that require treatment and respond to it [13]. Severe reactions are those that are potentially life threatening with impending death if not managed properly [2]. The severe allergic-like reactions include diffuse edema with dyspnea, diffuse erythema with hypotension, laryngeal edema with stridor, bronchospasms with hypoxia and anaphylactic shock. The severe physiologic reactions include vasovagal reactions resistant to treatment, convulsions, arrhythmia and hypertensive emergency [13]. The end result of severe allergic like and physiologic reactions is CPA which is a medical emergency and prompt and proper management using the BLS protocol and drugs including epinephrine, vasopressors, antihistamines and inhaled B-agonists is necessary to save lives.

Contrast induced acute kidney injury and nephropathy can also occur following contrast administration [19]. Risk factors include co morbidities like diabetes mellitus, dehydration, cardiac disease, hypertension and multiple iodinated contrast media doses in less than 24 hours. Baseline serum creatinine +/− glomerular filtration rate should be availed before injection of contrast media in at risk patients [13]. Contrast media administration in such patients can be done with caution by: reduced dose of contrast media, hydration and use of iso-osmolar agents.

5. Management of acute contrast media reactions

Management of acute contrast begins with discontinuation of injection if not completed [13, 20]. General principals of BLS and ACLS should apply in case of cardiorespiratory arrest.

Summary of the management of contrast reactions is as outlined in **Table 3** below.

6. Premedication of at risk patients

Premedication of patients who have a higher risk of acute allergic like reactions should be considered to reduce the chance of reaction occurrence [18]. For elective premedication oral prednisolone and diphenhydramine are used. For emergency premedication I.V methyl prednisolone sodium succinate or dexamethasone sodium sulfate. I.V diphenhydramine can be used instead of steroids in emergency cases [13].

7. Reaction rebound prevention

Intravenous corticosteroids play a role in preventing short term recurrence of an allergic like reactions. They may also be administered to patients having severe allergic like manifestations prior to transport to an emergency unit. They are however not useful in the acute treatment of any reaction.

Reaction	Monitoring	Treatment
Anaphylactoid		
Urticaria (skin rash)	Initial size with marking and follow	Mild-Usually none; if symptomatic consider diphenhydramine, 25–50 mg orally Moderate/Severe-monitor vitals and obtain IV access. Consider diphenhydramine, 25–50 mg orally intramuscularly/intravenously; epinephrine (1:1,000), 0.1–0.3 mL subcutaneously/intramuscularly
Bronchospasm	Oxygen saturation, pulse, Blood pressure (BP)	In all forms of bronchospasms: preserve IV access, monitor vitals and oxygen saturation and give oxygen by mask 6-10 L/min Mild: Inhaled B-agonist- 2 puffs at 90mcg/puff and can be repeated up to 3 times. If response is not satisfactory, emergency response team should be contacted. Moderate Inhaled B-agonist- 2 puffs at 90mcg/puff and can be repeated up to 3 times Epinephrine (1:1000), 0.3 mL intramuscularly-this can be repeated every 5-15 minutes as needed up to 1 ml(1 mg)total; OR Epinephrine (1:10,000), 1 mL(0.1 mg) intravenously (slowly) if hypotensive; This can be repeated every few minutes as needed up to 10 ml(1 mg) total call the emergency medical team; call the emergency medical team Severe: Epinephrine (1:1000), 0.1–0.3 mL intramuscularly-this can be repeated every 5-15 minutes as needed up to 1 ml(1 mg) total; OR Epinephrine (1:10,000), 1 mL(0.1 mg) intravenously (slowly) if hypotensive; This can be repeated every few minutes as needed up to 10 ml(1 mg) total Call the emergency medical team and Inhaled B-agonist (may work synergistically). Call the emergency medical team
Facial or laryngeal edema	Oxygen saturation, pulse, BP	In all forms of laryngeal edema: preserve IV access, monitor vitals and oxygen saturation and give oxygen by mask 6-10 L/min Call the emergency medical team if severe Epinephrine (1:1000), 0.3 mL intramuscularly-this can be repeated every 5-15 minutes as needed up to 1 ml(1 mg)total; OR Epinephrine (1:10,000), 1 mL(0.1 mg) intravenously (slowly) if hypotensive; This can be repeated every few minutes as needed up to 10 ml(1 mg) total call the emergency medical team
Hypotension(systolic BP <90 mmHg) and tachycardia (>100 bpm)	Oxygen saturation, pulse, BP	Preserve IV access, Elevate legs 60°; oxygen, 6–10 L/min; rapid intravenous fluids(1 liter of 0.9% normal saline or lactated Ringer's); epinephrine (1:10,000), 1 mL(0.1 mg) intravenously (slowly); This can be repeated every few minutes as needed up to 10 ml(1 mg) total OR Epinephrine (1:1000), 0.3 mL intramuscularly-this can be repeated every 5-15 minutes as needed up to 1 ml(1 mg)total call the emergency medical team
Hypotension(systolic BP <90 mmHg) and bradycardia (<60 bpm)	Oxygen saturation, pulse, BP	Elevate legs 60°; oxygen, 6–10 L/min; rapid intravenous fluids(1 liter of 0.9% normal saline or lactated Ringer's) If mild, no further treatment is necessary If patient remains symptomatic despite the above measures: Atropine, 0.6–1 mg intravenously (slowly); repeat to total of 2–3 mg (0.04 mg/kg) if needed; call the emergency medical team

Reaction	Monitoring	Treatment
Cardiac arrhythmia	Oxygen saturation, pulse, BP, ECG	Follow ACLS protocols; call the emergency medical team
Hypertensive crisis (diastolic BP >120 mmHg; systolic BP >200 mmHg)	Oxygen saturation, pulse, BP, ECG	Nitroglycerine, 0.4 mg sublingually; can repeat every 5-10 minutes OR Labetalol intravenously 20 mg, administer slowly over 2 minutes. The dose can be doubled every 10 minutes. OR Lasix intravenously 20-40 mg,slowly over 2 minutes. Phentolamine, 5 mg intravenously for pheochromocytoma; Call the emergency medical team
Seizures	Oxygen saturation, pulse, BP, ECG	Observe and protect the patient Secure airway; oxygen, 6–10 L/min; Preserve IV access and give diazepam, 5 mg intramuscularly/ intravenously OR midazolam, 0.5–1 mg intravenously OR phenytoin infusion, 15–18 mg/kg at 50 mg/min; call the emergency medical team
Hypoglycemia	Oxygen saturation, pulse, BP	If patient is able to swallow orally give half a cup of fruit juice or 15 g of glucose Is the patient is unable to swallow safely, obtain IV access and give 50% dextrose, 1 ampule-25gms over 2 minutes OR 100 ml/hr. of 5% dextrose. Is patient is unable to swallow and IV access is not available give intramuscular glucagon 1 mg.
Pulmonary edema	Oxygen saturation, pulse, BP, ECG	Preserve IV access, Secure airway; oxygen, 6–10 L/min; Elevate head of the bed furosemide, 20–40 mg intravenously (slowly over 2 minutes); morphine, 1–3 mg intravenously; call the emergency medical team

Table 3.
Management of contrast reactions.

7.1 Radiology department preparedness to manage anaphylactic reactions to contrast media

The hospital administration in liaison with the heads of the radiology department and the radiology contrast committee should set up and publish an institutional policy and procedure manual on contrast media administration.

The purpose of this manual is:

i. To ensure that administration of contrast media is done according to the protocols set up by the hospital and imaging department.

ii. To ensure that in case of adverse reactions to contrast media, appropriate steps are taken to manage them.

iii. To ensure that patients at risk of contrast media reactions or with prior history of such reactions receive appropriate premedication and are imaged using suitable protocols.

iv. To ensure that patients due to receive intravenous contrast media have appropriate laboratory tests done and reviewed by the radiologist to determine their suitability for the procedure.

Guidelines for administration on intravenous contrast:

i. Administration of intravenous contrast should be done by a trained radiology technician / nurse under the supervision of the radiologist and these staff should be competent in recognizing and managing an adverse reaction if it occurs.

ii. Standard operating procedures on the administration of intravenous contrast media should be set up and made available to the radiology clinical staff for reference when needed.

iii. The Radiologist should review all the imaging requests that require administration of intravenous contrast, to determine the protocol to be used which will depend on the patient's condition and clinical indication for the study.

iv. The radiology technician and nurse attending to the patient must take a detailed history on the current clinical condition, current medications, history of allergy, asthma and prior adverse reactions to drugs and contrast media.

v. If the patient is found to have risk factors or contraindications to administration of contrast media, then the radiologist will determine the protocol to be followed and premedication to be administrated if required.

vi. Protocols on the recognition and management of adverse reactions to contrast media should be set up and made available to all radiology clinical staff. These protocols ought to be illustrated in flow charts and placed in the various imaging sections in which intravenous contrast media is administered to facilitate proper management of these emergencies.

vii. Close liaison between the radiology department, the emergency response team and intensive care unit must be present to ensure that the radiology department will get adequate support in case of an emergency.

7.2 Radiology department emergency trolley

All imaging sections in the radiology department must be equipped with the emergency equipment and medication required to monitor and manage a patient in cardiopulmonary arrest and more specifically a patient undergoing a severe reaction to contrast media.

Majority of the emergency equipment and medication are part of the standard crash cart/ emergency trolley; therefore, it is upon the administration of the radiology department to decide whether a dedicated contrast reaction kit is necessary. This will depend on the size of the imaging department, patient numbers and budget allocations.

The basic equipment required to monitor patients experiencing an adverse reaction to contrast media include:

i. Devices for hemodynamic Monitoring-Pulse and blood pressure monitors.

ii. Devices for respiratory monitoring – Pulse oximeter.

iii. Body temperature monitor – Thermometer or adhesive pads with thermoelectric transducer.

iv. Blood glucose monitor.

v. Stethoscope.

Equipment and supplies for managing patients in an acute adverse reaction include:

i. Oxygen supply from a wall unit or oxygen cylinder.

ii. Devices to supply the supplemental oxygen e.g. nasal cannula, simple face mask, face mask with oxygen reservoirs (non-rebreather mask). The latter is preferred as it is able to deliver a large dose of approximately 95–100% oxygen at a flow rate of 10-15 ml/min. Another device is a bag mask device which uses positive pressure ventilation with a face mask or advanced airway to administer a high concentration of oxygen to the patient. These devices must be available in adult and pediatric sizes.

iii. Suction device used to clear the airway of secretions to enable the patient to breath. A patent airway is required for effective cardiopulmonary resuscitation in case of cardiopulmonary arrest in the case of severe contrast media reactions. The suction device may be wall mounted or mobile an I used in conjunction with suction tubing/ catheters.

Basic medication required in case of a contrast media reactions include:

i. Epinephrine

- Emergency trolley / crash carts in hospital setting are usually equipped in 1 mg in 10 ml of epinephrine for intravenous administration (1:10000).

- Epinephrine 1 mg in 1 ml vial is used for intramuscular injection.

- Epinephrine autoinjectors in pediatric, and adult doses can also be used if available.

ii. Oral and intravenous antihistamines.

iii. Inhaled or nebulized B2 agonists.

iv. Normal saline intravenous fluid in 500 ml and 1 liter bags/ bottles.

v. Atropine 1 mg in 10 ml for intravenous administration.

Additional medication and supplies include:

i. Emergency drugs – these include the standards emergency medications which are part of standard crash cart/ emergency trolley.

ii. Supplies that form part of the standard emergency trolley like various sizes of intravenous cannulas, needles, syringes and intravenous giving sets.

iii. Advanced cardiovascular life support equipment including:

- Advanced airway adjuncts e.g. endotracheal tube.
- Suction catheters.
- Automated external defibrillator.

In view that cardiopulmonary arrest and adverse reactions to contrast media in the radiology department are rare, it is imperative that periodic stock checks are done to ensure the equipment and medications stocked for the management of these emergencies are within the recommended validity period.

7.3 Hospital emergency response team

When faced with a severe reaction to contrast media in which the patient's condition warrants implementation of basic life support and advanced cardiac life support protocols, it is imperative that the hospital emergency response team be alerted to assist in initiation of these lifesaving protocols.

Modern radiology departments are fitted with an emergency bell that alerts the emergency response team to respond to an emergency in each imaging section. All radiology staff must be made aware of the location of these bells to activate them when needed.

In the event that such a system is not in place, the phone number of an internal/external emergency response unit should be clearly posted in each imaging section.

7.4 Training

Despite the rare occurrence of contrast media reactions, they may carry substantial morbidity and mortality and thus require immediate intervention by the attending staff. These staff must therefore be equipped with the knowledge and skills to initiate effective cardiopulmonary resuscitation in order to manage these emergencies as they await the arrival of the emergency response team.

All clinical staff should receive life support training upon employment and thereafter attend at least three yearly refresher course as recommended by the American heart association.

Continuous medical education on contrast media reactions and their management should be held frequently to ensure these vital knowledge and skills are up to date.

Advanced radiology life support ™ is a course that uses concepts from basic life support and advanced cardiac life support to radiology clinical staff on recognizing and managing life threatening emergencies occurring in the imaging department.

This training covers:

- Types of contrast media used in imaging.
- Recognition of the signs and symptoms of contrast media reactions.
- Risk factors of contrast induced nephropathy and approach to administration of contrast media in renal insufficiency.
- Safety of Gadolinium based contrast agents and nephrogenic systemic fibrosis.
- Airway management in emergencies.
- Safe management of sedated patients in the imaging department.

Advanced radiology life support ™ has been successful in United states of America and Canada in training of radiologists, radiology technicians and nurses in the management of contrast media reactions and cardiopulmonary arrest in the radiology department. Accreditation is by the Mayo clinic of medicine and Science.

This training is available online in form interactive videos, therefore imaging departments should allocate a budget for purchase of this training for each of its clinical staff members.

Author details

Callen Kwamboka Onyambu[1*], Angeline Anyona Aywak[1], Sarah Kemunto Osiemo[2] and Timothy Musila Mutala[1]

1 Department of Diagnostic Imaging and Radiation Medicine, University of Nairobi, Nairobi, Kenya

2 Kenyatta University Hospital, Nairobi, Kenya

*Address all correspondence to: callen.onyambu@uonbi.ac.ke

References

[1] Beckett KR, Moriarity AK, Langer JM. Safe use of contrast media: What the radiologist needs to know. Radiographics. 2015.

[2] Singh J, Daftary A. Iodinated contrast media and their adverse reactions. Journal of Nuclear Medicine Technology. 2008.

[3] Wang C.L., Cohan R.H., Ellis J.H., Caoili E.M., Wang G., Francis I.R. Frequency, outcome, and appropriateness of treatment of nonionic iodinated contrast media reactions. Am J Roentgenol. 2008;

[4] Gaeta TJ, Clark S, Pelletier AJ, Camargo CA. National study of US emergency department visits for acute allergic reactions, 1993 to 2004. Ann Allergy, Asthma Immunol. 2007;

[5] Osiem SK, Onyamb CK, Aywa AA. Knowledge and practices of cardiopulmonary arrest and anaphylactic reactions in the radiology department. South African J Radiol. 2020;

[6] Jung JW, Kang HR, Kim MH, Lee W, Min KU, Han MH, et al. Immediate hypersensitivity reaction to gadolinium-based MR contrast media. Radiology. 2012;

[7] Park HK, Kang MG, Yang MS, Jung JW, Cho SH, Kang HR. Epidemiology of drug-induced anaphylaxis in a tertiary hospital in Korea. Allergol Int. 2017;

[8] Katzberg RW, Haller C. Contrast-induced nephrotoxicity: Clinical landscape. Kidney Int. 2006;

[9] Katzberg RW. Urography into the 21st century: New contrast media, renal handling, imaging characteristics, and nephrotoxicity. Radiology. 1997.

[10] Cohan RH, Ellis JH. Iodinated contrast material in uroradiology: Choice of agent and management of complications. Urol Clin North Am. 1997;

[11] Tublin ME, Murphy ME, Tessler FN. Current concepts in contrast media-induced nephropathy. American Journal of Roentgenology. 1998.

[12] Mamoulakis C, Tsarouhas K, Fragkiadoulaki I, Heretis I, Wilks MF, Spandidos DA, et al. Contrast-induced nephropathy: Basic concepts, pathophysiological implications and prevention strategies. Pharmacology and Therapeutics. 2017.

[13] ACR Committee on drugs and contrast Media. ACR Contrast Manual v10.3. American College of Radiology. 2018.

[14] Almén T. The etiology of contrast medium reactions. Invest Radiol. 1994;

[15] Katzberg RW, Lamba R. Contrast-Induced Nephropathy after Intravenous Administration: Fact or Fiction? Radiologic Clinics of North America. 2009.

[16] Böhm I, Heverhagen JT, Klose KJ. Classification of acute and delayed contrast media-induced reactions: Proposal of a three-step system. Contrast Media Mol Imaging. 2012;

[17] J.M. EM, S. MB, R. MB, R. VC, A. A-L. Clinical characteristics of adverse reaction to iodinated contrast media. Allergy Eur J Allergy Clin Immunol. 2013;

[18] Dispenza MC, Ditto AM. Adverse Reactions to Contrast Media. In: Drug Allergy Testing. 2018.

[19] Hossain MA, Costanzo E, Cosentino J, Patel C, Qaisar H, Singh V,

et al. Contrast-induced nephropathy: Pathophysiology, risk factors, and prevention. Saudi journal of kidney diseases and transplantation : an official publication of the Saudi Center for Organ Transplantation, Saudi Arabia. 2018.

[20] Neumar RW, Shuster M, Callaway CW, Gent LM, Atkins DL, Bhanji F, et al. Part 1: Executive summary: 2015 American Heart Association guidelines update for cardiopulmonary resuscitation and emergency cardiovascular care. Circulation. 2015;